# THE COVID-19 GUIDEBOOK

## A BEGINNERS GUIDE TO EVERYTHING CORONAVIRUS RELATED

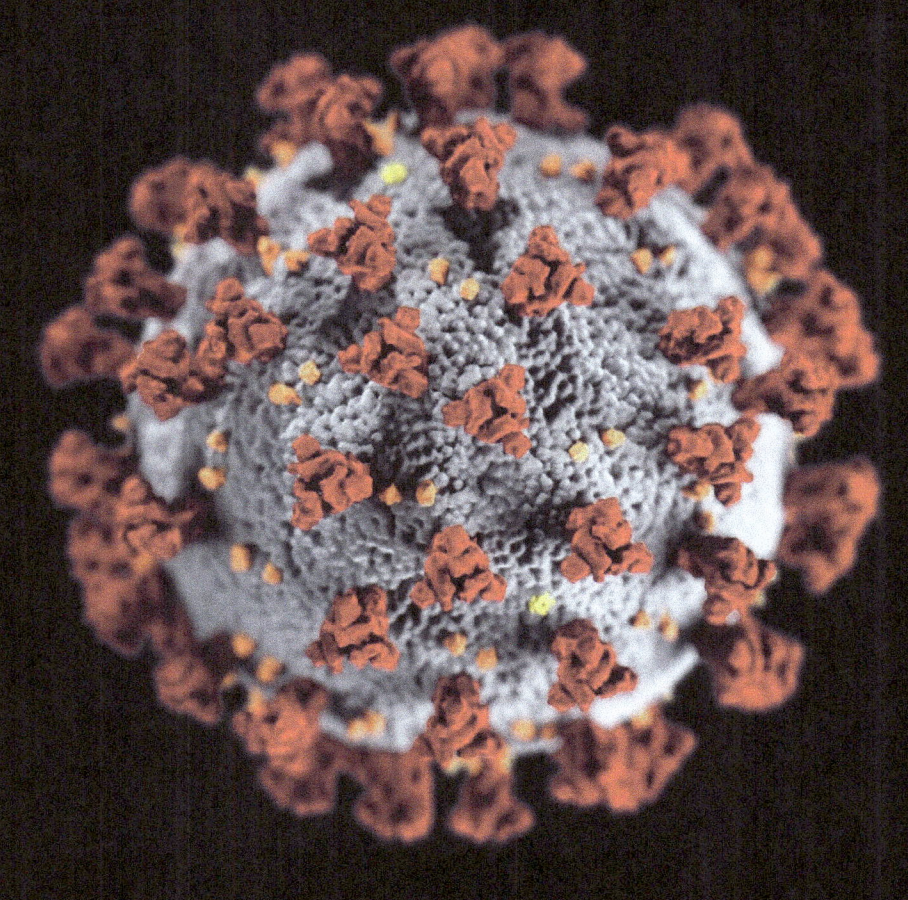

DR. ANDREW PIPER

# Contents

Foreword ..................................................................................................................... 4
What is the coronavirus? ............................................................................................. 5
What are different viral strains/variants/clades? ...................................................... 12
    How we track and name variants - Phylogenic trees ........................................ 13
    Mutations of interest .......................................................................................... 16
    N501Y (increased infectivity) ............................................................................. 16
    E484K (antibody evasion) ................................................................................... 16
Where does the coronavirus come from? .................................................................. 17
    The Wuhan Institute of Virology ......................................................................... 18
    The Huanan seafood wholesale market ............................................................. 20
    5G wireless networks ......................................................................................... 20
SARS-cov-2 infections ................................................................................................ 21
    How the immune system responds to a viral infection ..................................... 21
SARS-nCoV-2019 Symptoms and how to manage them ........................................... 26
    Inflammation ....................................................................................................... 26
    Fever .................................................................................................................... 27
    Dry cough ............................................................................................................ 28
    Tiredness ............................................................................................................. 28
    Less common symptoms .................................................................................... 29
    Aches and pains .................................................................................................. 29
    Diarrhoea ............................................................................................................ 29
    Conjunctivitis ...................................................................................................... 30
    Headaches .......................................................................................................... 30
    Loss of taste (Ageusia) and smell (Anosmia) ..................................................... 30
    Skin rash .............................................................................................................. 31
Rarer symptoms ......................................................................................................... 32
    Difficulty breathing ............................................................................................. 32
    Pneumonia .......................................................................................................... 33
    Chest pain or pressure ....................................................................................... 34
    Paralysis .............................................................................................................. 34
    Other symptoms ................................................................................................. 34
    Long corona ........................................................................................................ 35
How does the coronavirus spread? ........................................................................... 36
How can we stop the spread of the virus? ................................................................ 37
    Masks .................................................................................................................. 37

- Washing hands with soap or hand sanitizer ................................................................. 39
- Self-isolating and lockdowns ......................................................................................... 39
- Herd immunity ............................................................................................................... 42

## Testing for covid-19 .......................................................................................................... 44

### PCR tests ........................................................................................................................... 44
- The diagnostic pipeline ................................................................................................. 47
- The test kits ................................................................................................................... 47
- Swabbing (Nasopharyngeal swabs) ............................................................................. 49
- Logistics ......................................................................................................................... 51
- At the testing centre ..................................................................................................... 52
- Possible issues with PCR tests ..................................................................................... 53

### Antibody tests .................................................................................................................. 53

### SARS-cov-2 treatments ................................................................................................... 56
- Remdesivir ..................................................................................................................... 56
- Hydroxychloroquine ...................................................................................................... 58
- Drinking bleaches and disinfectant .............................................................................. 59
- Getting sunlight into people to destroy the virus ....................................................... 60
- Monoclonal antibody treatments ................................................................................. 61

### Vaccines ........................................................................................................................... 62
- Booster doses ................................................................................................................ 64
- How do we know if vaccines are safe and work before giving them to people? .... 64
- The current covid 19 vaccines on the market ............................................................ 67
- The Pfizer-BioNTech vaccine ........................................................................................ 67
- Pfizer BioNTech Phase 3 clinical trial data ................................................................. 69
- The Moderna vaccine .................................................................................................... 70
- Moderna vaccine phase 3 clinical trial data ............................................................... 71
- The Oxford-AstraZeneca vaccine .................................................................................. 71
- The Oxford-AstraZeneca phase 3 clinical trial data ................................................... 73
- How long will the vaccines protect us for? ................................................................. 74
- Controversy surrounding vaccines ............................................................................... 75

### Trends in the SARS-cov-2 cases ..................................................................................... 78
- Seasonal trends ............................................................................................................. 78
- Age and gender ............................................................................................................. 78
- Race ................................................................................................................................ 79
- How dangerous is covid-19 .......................................................................................... 79
- When will life return to normal? ................................................................................. 80

    The positive impact of the pandemic ................................................................................ 81
Appendix ............................................................................................................................. 82
    Covid-19 genome ............................................................................................................. 82
    Spike protein amino acid sequence ................................................................................ 90

# Foreword

Since the covid-19 virus was first detected in human beings in November 2019, the world as we know it has changed beyond all comprehension. Words that were once considered scientific jargon have now become commonplace in our lives. In a world filled with "fake news" and contradictory statements and policies from the powers that be, how do we know who to trust and what to believe? It is the purpose of this book to cut through the mire and try to explain the coronavirus pandemic in a way that is easy to understand. To try and frame the most important historical event in our lifetimes in a clear and concise manner. But how can I ask you, the reader, to trust me, the author, without first explaining who I am and where my knowledge of the coronavirus pandemic comes from. My name is Dr Andrew Piper, I have a Master´s degree in Medicinal and Biological Chemistry and a PhD in Biosensor development, both from the University of Edinburgh. What are "Biosensors" you ask? Quite simply they are devices that detect something biological, usually (but not exclusively) detecting something within a person that makes them sick. The best examples of Biosensors are probably pregnancy tests, which detect the hormones in a woman´s urine that are only present when she is pregnant, or blood glucometers, those little devices you may have seen diabetics use to measure the sugar levels in their blood. To put it another way, my job is to develop new (or improve existing) diagnostic tests. Since completing my PhD I have held a number of post-doctoral jobs (short term research positions) at universities around the world. These have included working on a blood test for Parkinson´s disease at the University of Oxford and developing wearable sensors to analyse sweat at the KTH Royal institute of technology in Stockholm. It was while I was living in Stockholm that the coronavirus was declared a pandemic by the world health organisation (WHO) in February of 2020. In March, an email found its way into my inbox asking for academics with relevant experience to help establish and run a "national pandemic response centre" at the Karolinska Institute (Stockholm´s University hospital). Since April I have been involved in the setting up and day to day running of a RT-qPCR lab responsible for the testing of over 600 000 patient samples. I mention this only to give myself some credibility in your eyes when it comes to the contents of this book.

From a personal viewpoint, in November 2020 I myself contract the corona virus, most probably from the public transport network in Stockholm. So can speak from personal experience about how the virus feels and progresses. Likewise, I have known several family members and close friends who have come down with coronavirus and know the feelings of worry that go through us all when those we care about get sick. Most people quite rightly have a lot of questions and concerns over the current situation. While the media and politicians are constantly rattling on about "R numbers", "variants of the virus", "antibodies", "PCR tests", etc. It struck me through having conversations with family and friends that the vast majority of people have no idea what most of these terms mean. Most of it is technical jargon. More worryingly, watching the news it becomes apparent very quickly that most of the journalists and politicians discussing the pandemic don´t have the faintest clue about any of this stuff either. I therefore thought there was the need for a relatively short and easy to understand book that could educate the general reader, and maybe even some advanced readers, about the more important aspects of the coronavirus. So if you are wondering what this virus actually is? How vaccines work? Why do we need to wear masks and do they really stop the virus spreading? Or anything else covid related, I hope that you will take the time to read and hopefully even enjoy this book.

## What is the coronavirus?

So perhaps it is best to start from the very beginning, what exactly is a virus? In the simplest terms you can think of a virus as a very small parcel of genetic material. Their sole purpose is to get into suitable living cells and hijack their machinery to make lots of copies of themselves, that can then go and infect other host cells. In principle they can be thought of as parasites, unable to do anything by themselves and relying entirely on their hosts to be able to flourish. We all know people like this. Whilst this sounds pretty simple, the explanation given can be broken down and expanded upon.

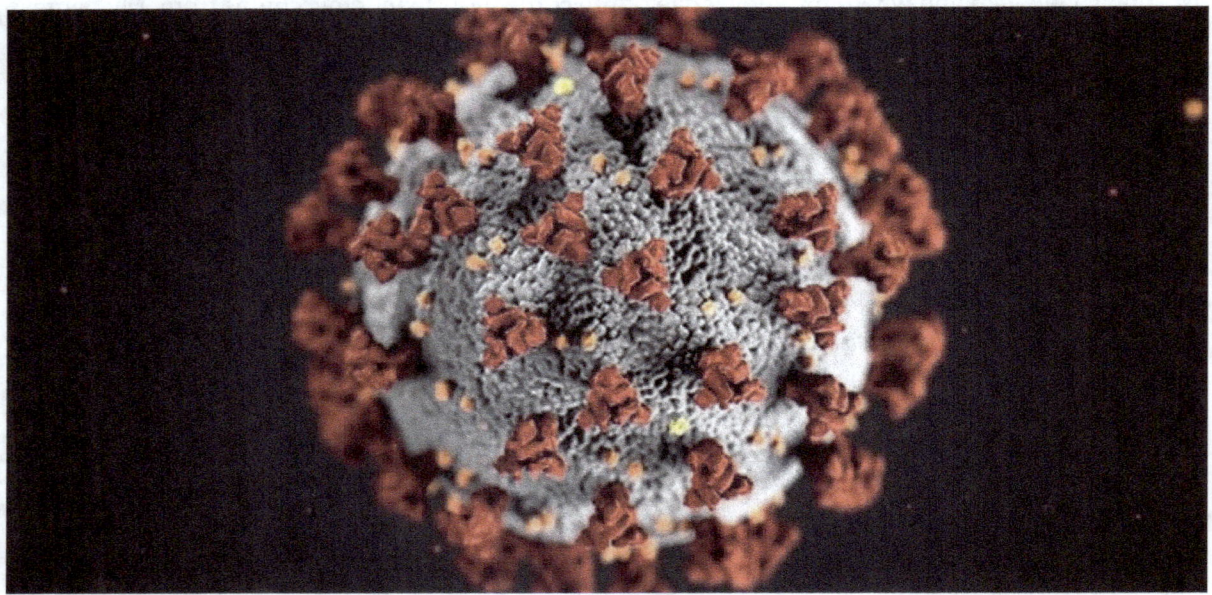

In order to properly describe what a virus is and how it goes about its business, we need to understand its structure. As with so many things in biology, the structure gives it function. An important distinction to get right at this point is the difference between a virus and virion. When referring to the virus we are speaking about lots of virions of the same type, many covid-19 virions. A virion is one singular virus entity, such as shown in the image above. Viruses refers to lots of viruses of different types, e.g. corona and HIV. Most virions are tens of nanometres to hundreds of nanometres in diameter, for scale one nanometre is what you would get if you divided a single millimetre into one million equally sized pieces. To be honest, it is not possible for the human brain to comprehend what that actually means, at least not most people´s brains. How can anyone look at a 1 mm marking on a ruler and imagine it divided into a million little pieces? Personally I have always like to think of things in relation to one another to comprehend their sizes. Everything in the world is built out of atoms. Atoms are usually 0.05 – 0.5 nm in diameter, with most of the common ones used in nature at the lower end of that scale. The coronavirus is about 50 to 200 nm in diameter. So the virus is as wide as 100 to 4000 atoms lined up perfectly next to each other like marbles. Most of the living cells that comprise every form of life however are 1 000 to 100 000 nm (1 – 100 micrometres) long. Much larger than viruses but still microscopic too us, in fact, most viruses are too small to even be seen under a normal light microscope and special techniques are required to image them.

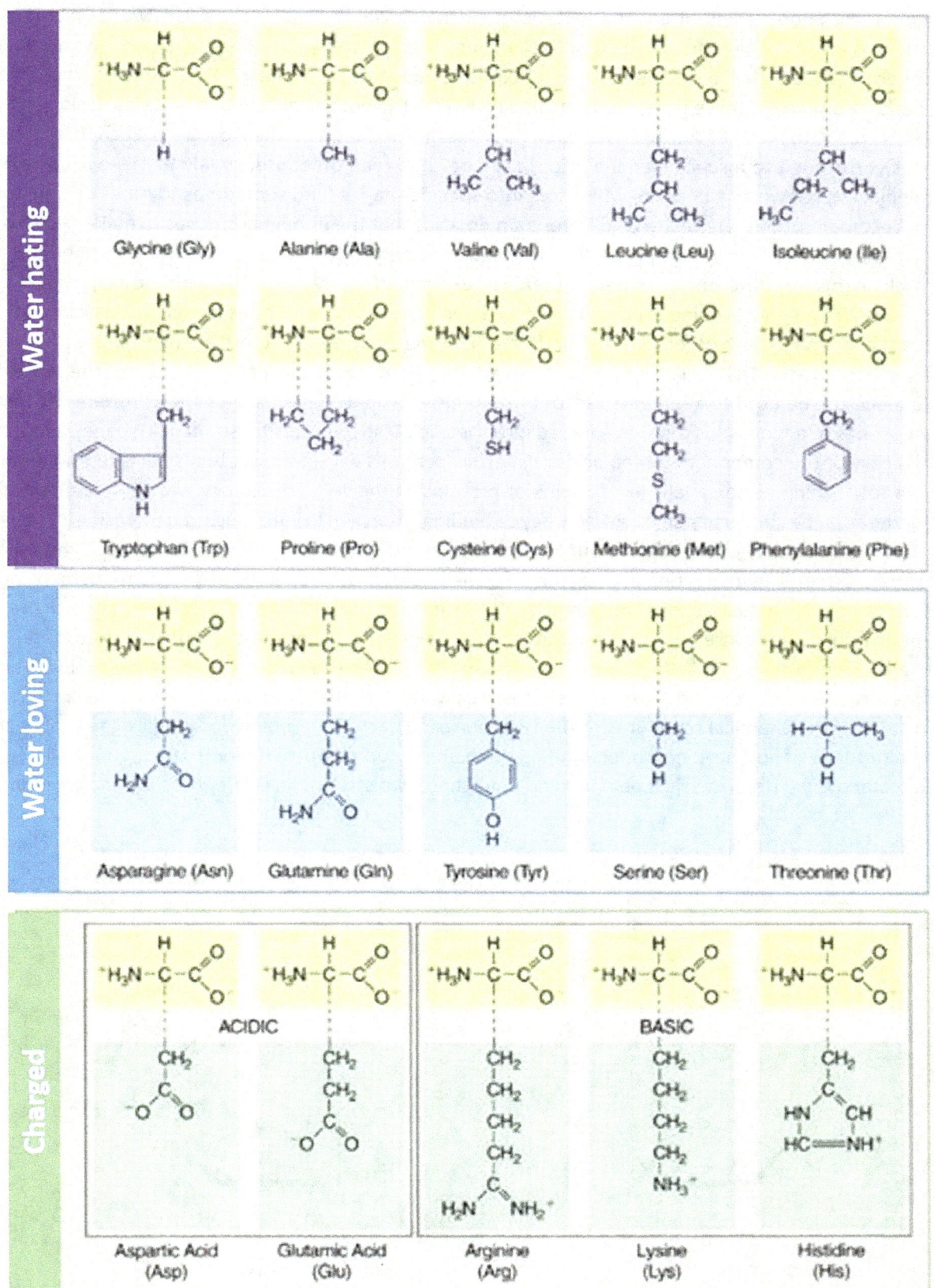

When most people think of genetic material their minds will instantly spring to DNA (deoxyribose nucleic acid). Anyone who did high school biology will probably be able to tell you with some confidence that DNA is a double helix with "bases" of adenine, thymine, cytosine and guanine; and that the sequence of these bases forms a large code that the body uses to make proteins. Inside cells, DNA is "read" to make RNA (ribose nucleic acid) which is then used to make proteins. Each three RNA bases correspond to a specific amino acid, these are then read off consecutively to make a string of amino acids, known as a peptide, which fold into specific shapes (and sometimes to other chemicals) and become proteins. There are 20 different amino acids that the human body uses to make proteins. Their chemical structures and properties are shown in the picture above. The different amino acids are all chemically different from each other. For example, they can be salts with either positive or negative charge, these amino acids will prefer to be in water and their opposite charges in a chain will attract and bind to each other to form bonds in a 3D structure. Likewise, there are hydrophobic (water hating) amino acids that will prefer to be in oily environments, a lot of these in one part of the protein sequence can be used to keep that part of the protein in a lipid bilayer (see below). Proteins are just long strings of amino acids that have folded into specific 3D shapes, it is these specific shapes and the chemistry of the component amino acids in specific locations within the protein structure that allow them to do things. I personally like to think of proteins as the verbs of biology, always doing things. Whether that be converting sugar into energy or binding to oxygen in your lungs and releasing it where it is needed; virtually everything in your body that is "done", is done by a protein. If we continue the metaphor, DNA is an instruction manual for life, RNA is someone reading the instructions out loud and proteins are the actual actions described being performed. Now some viruses have, like us, their genetic information stored as DNA. A lot of them, the coronavirus included, do not. They store their genetic information as RNA, these viruses are collectively called retroviruses. You are probably at this point wondering what exactly RNA is. Well, chemically, it is not that different to DNA. I have included a picture of the chemical structures of the two alongside each other below for a quick game of spot the difference. If you have no understanding of chemistry don't worry it won't affect your ability to understand the differences, just bear in mind that where two straight lines join there is a carbon atom.

DNA-thymine                                             RNA-Uracil

The two main differences between RNA and DNA are that there is, firstly, an extra oxygen on the bottom right carbon in the 5-carbon ring. It is the lack of this oxygen that gives DNA its name DEOXYribose nucleic acid rather than ribose nucleic acid. The "deoxy" literally refers to the lack of an oxygen in the chemical structure. The second difference between DNA and RNA is that rather than one of the bases being thymine, RNA uses a similar base called "Uracil" instead. This has one less methyl group (A carbon with three hydrogen atoms) in its structure; as can be seen in the structures provided. Whilst these differences may not sound like much, the physical differences between RNA and DNA are quite pronounced. RNA is a lot less stable than DNA, mainly due to the presence of this oxygen. When I say it is less stable I mean it degrades much faster. Importantly, RNA is more prone to mutations than DNA, which means that retroviruses evolve much faster than DNA viruses. This allows them to adapt and change very quickly which makes them very difficult to treat or vaccinate for. However, it is not impossible. For example, the polio virus is a retrovirus for which several working vaccines exists. To continue with the metaphor from before, DNA is like writing down the instructions to life on a piece of paper, RNA is like passing it on through word of mouth. The general gist can be passed on but is more prone to errors and changes over time, often being adapted to make the story more engaging to the readers of the day. The core concept of all biology is that DNA, makes RNA, makes proteins. Without this, life as we know it would not exist. Even when we look for life on other planets we are looking for DNA, RNA or proteins on those planets.

A virus has a very simple life cycle, compared to you and me. All it needs to do is gain entry into a host cell and hijack it to make more copies of itself. You, on the other hand, have the genetic code to make all the different types of cells in your body stored in every cell. As such, viral genomes (their entire DNA sequence) are much smaller than our own. The 2019-coronavirus has a genome that is just under 30 000 base pairs long, if you are interested it can be found in the appendix of this book. In contrast, each of your cells contains your genetic sequence which is 3 100 000 000 bases long. Whilst the coronavirus genetic sequence is small compared to yours, coronaviruses in general have the largest genomes of any retrovirus. However, the size of the genome is actually not that important biologically, a larger genome does not correlate to a more complex life form. In fact, the animal with the largest genome in the world is the Australian lungfish, with a genome 150 000 000 000 bases long, about 50 times larger than our own. This does not mean that a lungfish is 50 times more advanced than you or me, all it means is that each of its cells contains more DNA than each of our cells.

So we know that the coronavirus is a very small parcel of RNA that is trying to find a host cell to make more copies of itself, but just what is this "parcel"? Technically known as a "capsid", the coronavirus envelope in which the viral RNA is contained is comprised of a lipid membrane and some proteins. A lipid membrane is made by two layers of "lipids", molecules that are often drawn as little balls with two long tails, see image below, the tails are very oily so will try to stay away from water, but the heads are salty and will happily sit in water. What normally happens to molecules like this is the form what are called micelles, spheres where the molecules can arrange themselves to keep the oily parts together and the salty heads facing the water on the inside and outside of the micelle. This is essentially the structure of all mammalian cells, where you have water inside and out.

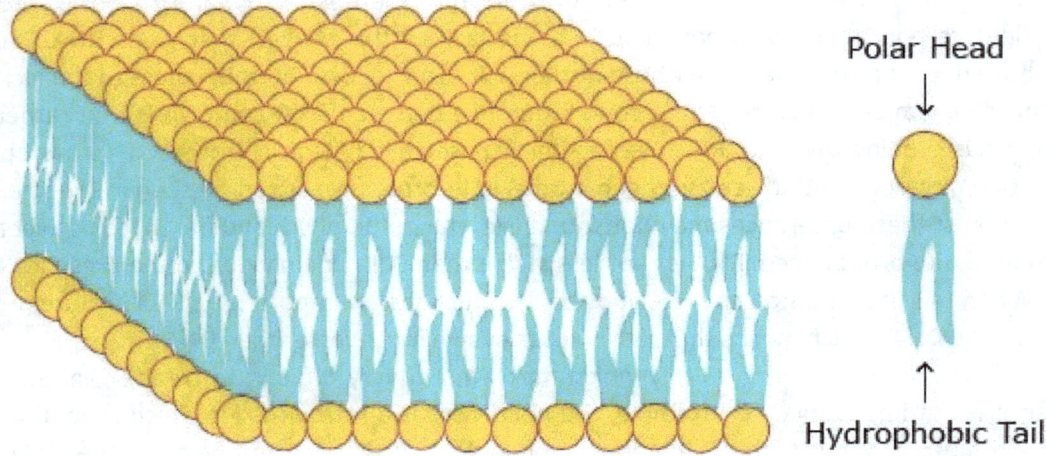

Lots of viruses and cells have lipid bilayers, the things that make them unique and give them function are their proteins. The corona virus has four different types of proteins labelled as N, M, E and S in the picture below. Each of these proteins plays a key role in how the virus operates and survives so will be discussed in more detail.

The first protein we will look at is the nucleocapsid proteins, labelled as (N) in the picture below. These are within the lipid bilayer (blue in the picture) and bind to the RNA. The N proteins in coronaviruses are what are known as multifunctional proteins, as they perform several functions.

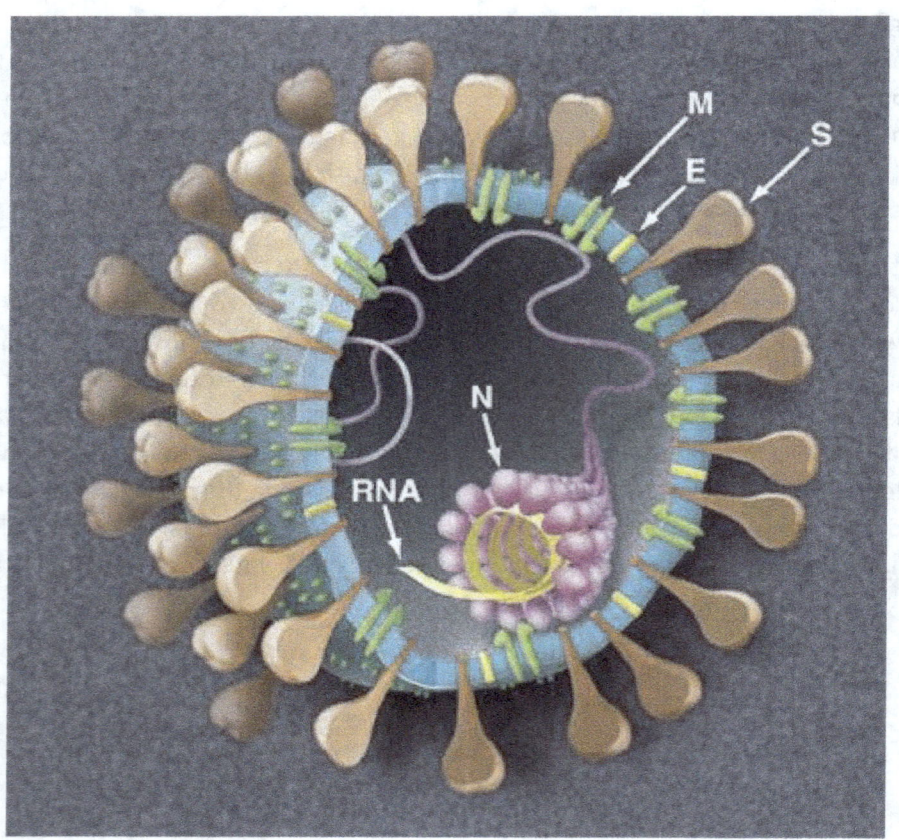

Whilst research into the cov-19 virus is still ongoing and the exact function of all the proteins are not known, it is safe to assume that the N proteins in this coronavirus perform similar function to those in other coronaviruses. The N protein in other coronaviruses is known to: stabilise RNA, help with the replication of the virus, disrupt host cells, disrupt the host immune system and cause cell apoptosis (a process by which cells that think they are unhealthy or dangerous commit suicide). In other word's these proteins can actively cause your immune cells to kill themselves, increasing the viruses chance of survival.

The "M" proteins (Membrane proteins) are embedded within the membranes and help define and control the structure and shape of the virus. Everything from the curvature and rigidity of the capsid to the distribution and clustering of the other membrane proteins (E and S) is controlled by the M proteins. They also play key roles in the formation of the virus within the host cells.

The "E" proteins are envelope proteins, so called because they are predominantly involved in the formation of new virus particles within the host cells. Sounds pretty similar to the M proteins right? The E proteins help the M proteins and in some coronaviruses, if they are removed they viruses still survive and replicate, although will not be as "healthy" as they would be if the E proteins were present. Effectively leading to crippled viruses. E proteins are also multifunctional proteins and have been shown to be involved in the release of virions from the host cells and in some cases can even be involved in disease pathogenesis (the way in which the virus makes you sick).

The S proteins are so labelled as they are known as "Spike" proteins. These are the ones that are discussed most in the news and are key to finding vaccines and treatments for the virus. These spike proteins have a portion, let's say their feet, that are quite oily so anchor the proteins into the lipid membrane, and a water loving sticky out bit that stick out of the virus and allow it to attach to host cells. The flu virus has two spike proteins: hemagglutinin (H) and neuraminidase (N). At the time of writing there are 18 different subtypes of the hemagglutinin protein (H1 to H18) and 11 neuraminidase (N1 to N11) subtypes that have been observed in nature. You might have heard of people referring to swine flu as H1N1 or bird flu as H5N1. This basically just means that those pandemics were the influenza virus with those specific subtypes of spike protein. So what is the difference between the subtypes? It can be as small as a single amino acid in the protein chain being changed to something different, such changes happen routinely and only require a single base in the genomic sequence to be miscopied as a different one, I explain how mutations arise in section xx below. Most of the time these changes have no effect but occasionally they can make the virus much more deadly or contagious, such as the Spanish influenza (H1N1) which between 1918-1920 was responsible for the death of an estimated 50-100 million people.

The cov-19 virus only has one spike protein, although this has mutated to form many new variants. The cov-19 spike protein has two component parts the S1 unit and the S2 unit. Each unit is a separate amino acid chain that then get stuck together to form the spike protein. The S1 unit can be thought of like a glove, that will only fit specific hand shaped proteins of the right size and shape on the host cells the virus can infect. The second subunit (S2) drives the merging of the virus capsid with the host cell membrane. The S1 unit has a specific shape and chemical structure that allows it to bind to the host cell it is going to infect. It is this protein and mutations in it that are responsible for the virus being able to infect cells. If the protein mutates to a form that has a higher chance of binding to your cells, then the infectivity of the virus goes up. When you are infected with the virus your body will produce antibodies to fight the infection which bind specifically to this S protein. When vaccines are developed they are designed to mimic this protein to teach your immune system how to recognise and fight off the virus. This protein is what allows the virus to not only infect specific species but determines which cells within your body the virus can infect. In other words, it determines whether the virus will infect your brain, your lungs or your liver. As far as most of us are concerned, the S protein is by far the most important protein in the virus.

This brings us quite neatly onto viral replication. How does a virus go about creating more of itself? The first step is that the virus needs to come into contact with a suitable host cell. The spike protein of the covid-19 protein binds to angiotensin-converting enzyme 2 (ACE2) receptors. These ACE2 receptors are proteins that can be found on the outside of human lung, heart, kidney, artery, intestine and liver cells. Enzymes are just proteins that "catalyse" (speed up or initiate) chemical reactions, and are conveniently named after the reactions that they catalyse. ACE1 (normally just called ACE) converts angiotensin-1 to angiotensin-2 and ACE2 converts angiotensin-2 back to angiotensin 1. Angiotensin-1 is a short chain of amino acids that acts as a "vasodilator", it causes your veins and arteries to expand, which reduces your blood pressure; whereas angiotensin 2 is a "vasoconstrictor", causing your veins and arteries to tighten and increase your blood pressure. The ACE-2 receptors are particularly abundant in your lungs, which makes them ideal receptors for an airborne virus like the coronavirus to bind to. When you breath in air with covid-19 virions in it, they will naturally be drawn into your lungs where they can come into contact with, and bind to, these ACE2 receptors.

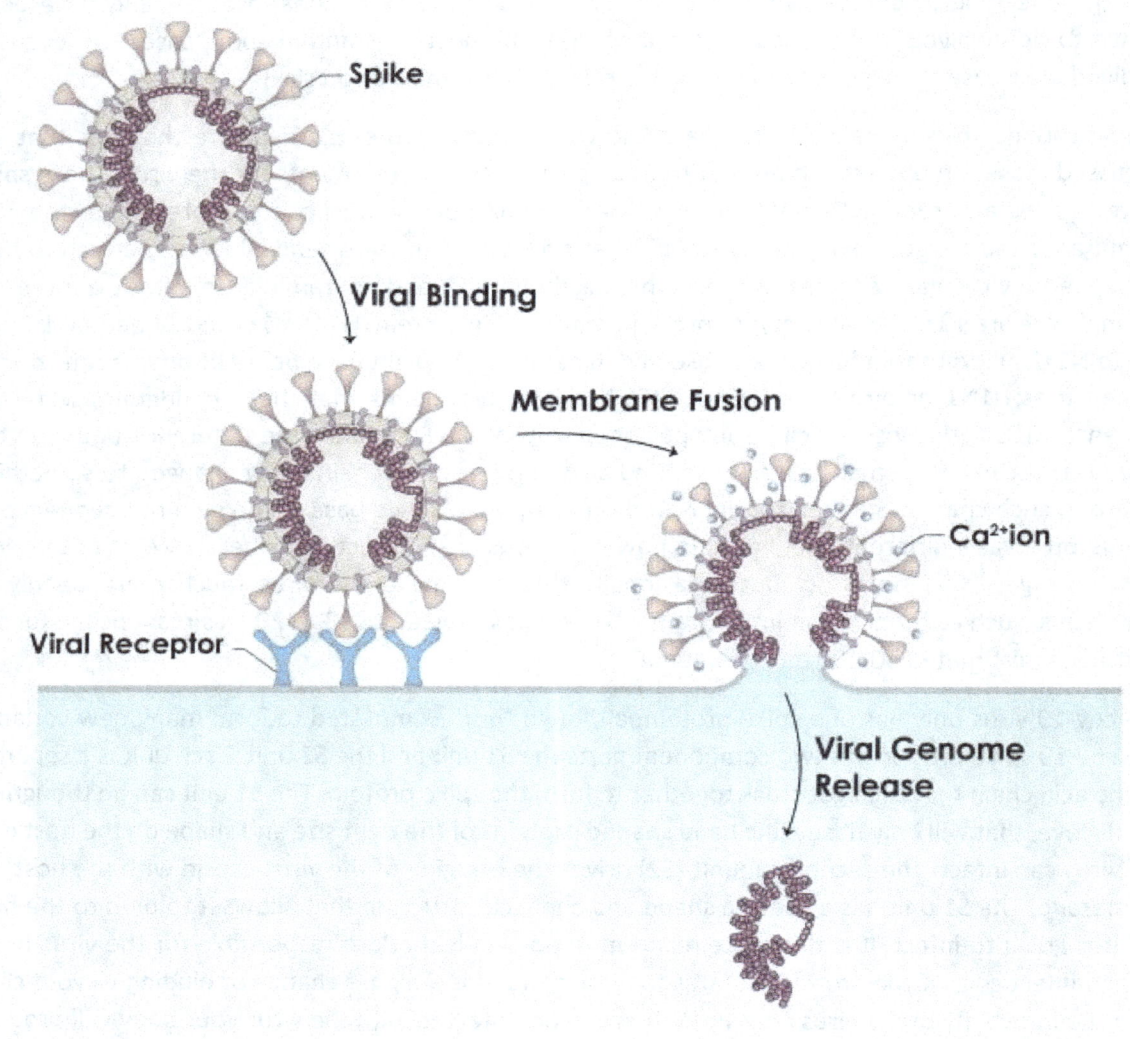

Once the spike protein has bound to the ACE2 receptor, the viral envelope is brought into contact with the cell membrane, the lipid bilayer of the host cell and the virus merge and the viral RNA is released into the host cell. The RNA is then transported to the cell nucleus when it is converted to DNA. This DNA encodes instructions on how to make new viruses and your host cell starts to work tirelessly to produce copies of the virus. On average each infected cell will produce about 1000 virions before they burst and release the virus. These virions can then go on to infect nearby cells, get transported around the body spreading the infection to other organs or get released back into the world where they can infect other people. It takes roughly 10 minutes to go from the spike protein binding to the ACE2 receptor to the viral RNA being released into the host cell and the cell will usually burst, releasing virions, after about 10 hours.

## What are different viral strains/variants/clades?

The terms strains, variants and clades are used interchangeably, but the technically correct term is clade. Clades are defined as a group of organisms that have a single common ancestor. Much like siblings, they are genetically different; but their genetic sequences can all be traced back to their parents. The cov-19 virus is constantly mutating. Mutations are caused by random mistakes when the RNA is being copied in the host cell. This can change a sequence that was originally AAA to something like ACA, ATA, or AGA, or maybe even adding an extra base where there was none before (e.g. AAAA, AATA, AACA, AAGA) or missing out a base by mistake (AA). These are termed substitutions, when the wrong base is put in; deletions, when a based is missed out; or additions, when an extra base is added. Since a sequence of three bases codes for a specific amino acid, when a substitution occurs, one of the amino acids in a protein will be changed. Sometimes this can cause a large, crucial change, other times it has very little or no effect at all. When insertions or deletions occur, not only the amino acid where the mutation has arisen changes, but all the subsequent amino acids in the protein chain are changed. These types of mutations are much more severe and usually result in proteins that do not work and that virus will normally die off. Because mutations are so dangerous, most of the DNA/RNA in every genome on the planet is "junk DNA" think of it this way, if you are going to have 1 mutation in every new virus made, it makes sense to have 99% of the DNA just filler that doesn't code for any proteins at all. That way when mutations occur they are usually in the part of the genetic sequence that doesn't matter, but the sequence that code for all your proteins is preserved. Although from time to time, the mutation will, by complete chance, happen where you don't want it. When the spike protein sequence has a substitution in one of the RNA bases, the amino acid change can prevent your immune cells from recognising it. Mutations in the virus can change the lethality and transmissibility of the virus, but they can also render vaccines useless, stop PCR and antibody tests from working, re-infect people who have recovered from a previous variant and allow the virus to evade different antiviral drugs. The more people that have the virus, the more cells that there will be actively copying the viral RNA, which increases the number of mutations and therefore variants. In other words, the more people who have the virus the more mutations will occur. There are currently hundreds of known variants of the covid-19 virus.

|  | Original | Substitution | Deletion | Addition |
|---|---|---|---|---|
| **DNA** | AAATTTCCCGGG | AAAT**C**TCCCGGG | AA_TTTCCCGGG | AAA**C**TTTCCCGGG |
| **RNA** | UUUAAAGGGCCC | UUUA**G**AGGGCCC | UU_AAAGGGCCC | UUU**G**AAAGGGCCC |
| **Amino acid** | Phe-Lys-Gly-Pro | Phe-**Arg**-Gly-Pro | **Leu**-Lys-Gly-Pro | Phe-**Glu-Arg-Gly** |

## How we track and name variants - Phylogenic trees

A Phylogenic tree is basically a family tree for the virus. We can track mutations and assign names for specific variants based on where they fall on the phylogenic tree. Every time there is a mutation the tree splits with the original still existing and multiplying alongside the new strain. These graphs have time going along the bottom, which allows us to track the evolution of the different strains. When we look at the phylogenic tree for the covid-19 virus it gives us some idea of how quickly the virus mutates. We very quickly go from one initial virus to hundreds of variants within a year. You can also notice that some branches of the tree have mutated more than others. This typically means that one of the earlier mutations has made that strain more contagious. The more people that have the virus, the more virions that are being made and the greater the chance of further mutations.

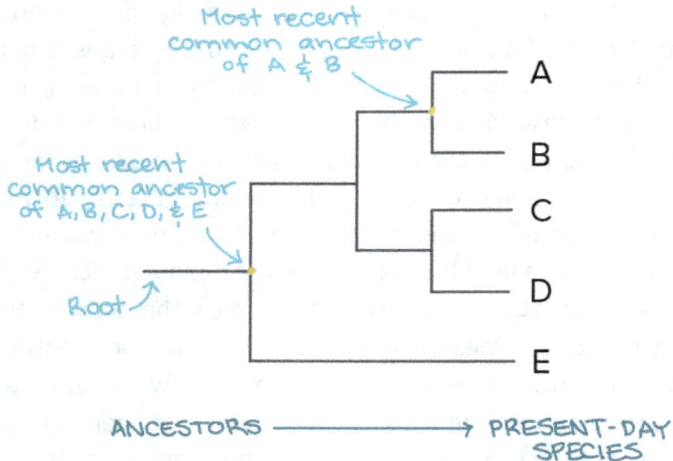

When it comes to naming variants, this is currently done by referring to the country in which they were first identified and their position on the phylogenic tree. For example, let us look at the B.1.1.7. variant, also known as the British or London variant. This clade was first spotted in London in September of 2020. By November it accounted for 40-80% of all the cases in London; as this variant is far more infectious than the original and earlier covid-19 clades. The "B" in the name comes from the fact that this clade was first identified in Britain, and the 1.1.7. can be followed on the phylogenic tree to find the exact mutations and origins of this clade. There are currently efforts being made to change this naming system. There are several reasons for this, the first is that some governments are unwilling to report new clades that originate in their countries. Personally I don't think that removing their country from the name will combat this. The stigma will arise regardless. Colloquially people will always refer to them as the British strain, or the Brazilian strain. However, if people understood that these mutations arise completely by chance; no strain is worse because of the country it originates in. Mutations happen everywhere and everywhere all the time. The fact that one specific mutation arises in a country has nothing to do with the country it arises in. It is a completely random process and no stigma should be attached to the emergence of new variations.

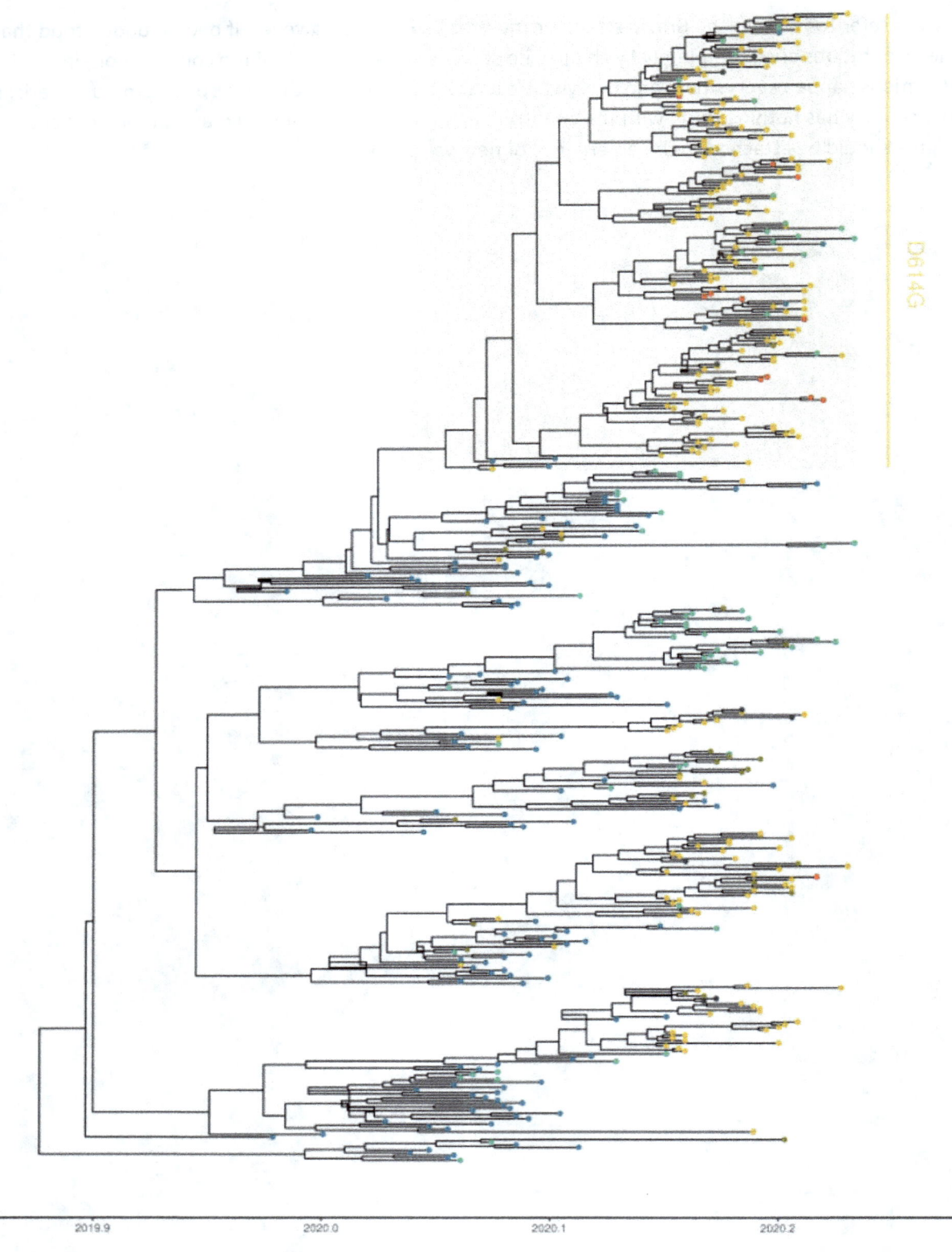

Thankfully the naming system for specific mutations in a protein are much easier to understand. To do this we need to build upon our knowledge of proteins, which are, as you will recall, long chains of amino acids. There are 20 naturally occurring amino acids, so biologists assigned each of them a letter of the alphabet. When a substitution mutation occurs within a protein, we are interested in knowing what the original amino acid was, where in the chain this has happened and what the new amino acid is. An example of this is the N501Y variant, where the amino acid asparagine (N) was the 501st amino acid in the protein chain, but has now changed to tyrosine (Y). How exactly does changing one amino acid for another actually affect the virus?

## Mutations of interest

As you can see from the phylogenic tree, there are far too many different clades to be able to discuss them all properly, but I have picked a few mutations to discuss in a little more detail to discuss how they change the virus. These are not the only mutations that can change the properties of the virus but are nice examples of how the process works

## N501Y (increased infectivity)

Genetically the three base RNA sequence that codes for asparagine (N) is "AAC", the code for tyrosine is "UAC". So in this variant, the first "A" has been miscopied as a "U", the amino acid changed and now the protein chain is different. This specific amino acid (asparagine) is directly responsible for chemically binding to the host cell ACE2 receptor. Whilst asparagine binds to the receptor, tyrosine forms an even stronger bond. This means the virus is less likely to fall off or not bind properly and infect the host cell. As a result, this mutation makes the virus more infectious than the earlier version with asparagine at position 501 in the spike protein. That is how one simple chance misreading can make a virus more infectious.

## E484K (antibody evasion)

In this mutation an aspartic acid (E) has been replaced with a lysine (K), studies have found that most of the antibodies that people who have had the virus make will bind (at least partially) to the aspartic acid at position 484 in the spike protein. Lysine is chemically very different to aspartic acid so the antibodies that the immune system has developed will not work against this variant of the virus. People who had an earlier form of the virus can get SARS-cov-2 again if they are re-infected by a variant with this mutation. Likewise, the vaccines that are on the market are training the immune system for a spike protein with aspartic acid at position 484, so there is a chance that if your immune system makes antibodies that bind to that part of the virus, the vaccine might not protect you from future infection against this mutation. Remember that everybody makes different antibodies so there is a chance that if you are vaccinated or have recovered from an infection of the earlier variant your antibodies bind in a different part of the spike protein (not on position 484). In this case you will still have an immunity to the new form of the virus. Studies show that in about 70% of people who develop antibodies and T cells (whether naturally or through vaccination), the antibodies and T cells they make will bind to the aspartic acid at position 484. Unfortunately, this means that this variant will be able to re-infect about 70% of people who have recovered from an earlier infection or been vaccinated.

## The Delta Variant

Technically known as the B.1.617.2. variant, this variant was first identified in India in December of 2020. Since then it has been found in many European countries, most predominantly the U.K. where it is now the most prevalent strain. It is now also the most prevalent cause of new cases in the U.S.A. this variant is almost twice as infectious as the original covid-19 virus. The initial data seems to suggest that most of the vaccines still work against this variant. Given how rapidly it is spreading it is not unreasonable to assume that this will be the most widespread and dominant variant of the virus in 2021.

## Where does the coronavirus come from?

In some ways this is the easiest and in other ways the hardest of questions to answer. I will start off by saying what we know for certain before going into some of the conspiracy theories about the virus.

This is not the only coronavirus, in fact there are about a dozen different coronaviruses, several of which have infected people before. Most notably SARS-coV and MERS-coV which are acronyms of the Severe Acute Respiratory Syndrome coronavirus and the Middle Eastern Respiratory Syndrome coronavirus respectively. The SARS-coV virus was responsible for an outbreak between 2002 and 2004 which infected 8 442 and killed a reported 774 people in 29 countries around the world. This virus originated from bats in China and spread to the human population killing 11% of those it infected. Like covid-19 it infected the lungs and symptoms of both virus types are very similar, including:

- High fever (>38 °C, 100 F)
- Coughing
- Difficulty breathing
- Muscle pains
- Tiredness
- Cough
- Sore throat
- Pneumonia

As with SARS-cov-2 (the disease caused by covid-19), not everyone who got SARS-coV got the same symptoms. Overall the SARS-coV was not able to spread as much as the cov-19 coronavirus, but was more deadly, according to the available data.

The Middle Eastern Respiratory Syndrome coronavirus was first identified in Saudi Arabia in 2012 and is still active today. Also thought to have originated from bats the virus is believed to have jumped to camels before being transmitted to people. To date (2021) there have been about 2 500 reported cases of MERS which kills about 35% (866 total deaths) of those who it infects; making it the most fatal of the coronaviruses to have infected people. Luckily this virus has difficult in going from one person to another, with the majority of cases occurring in people who have come into close contact with camels that are sick with the virus. The symptoms are again similar to those of SARS-coV and SARS-coV-2. There have been two distinct outbreaks of the MERS-coV: in Saudi Arabia in 2014 and South Korea in 2015. With hindsight we should have been more prepared and worried about a coronavirus pandemic, the warning signs were there, but the scale of the current pandemic has taken the whole world by surprise.

Like SARS-coV and MERS-coV, the cov-19 virus originated in bats. In this instance the first human transmission recorded was in the Wuhan province of China in November of 2019. How do we know that these viruses originated in bats? Well for starters, bats are known to host a variety of coronaviruses, so they are a good place to start looking. Secondly, when the virus was first detected, its genome was "sequenced", its entire genetic code was figured out. Once the sequence is known it can be compared to the genomes of all other sequenced viruses stored on a database. Then the similarity of the viral genome to other genomes in the database is ranked. This coronavirus (cov-19) was found to be most similar (96.2% identical) to that of a coronavirus discovered in bats in south China in 2012. Making it the most likely source of a virus that mutated to be able to infect humans.

Once it got into a human host it seems to have been able to spread rapidly and is fatal in about 4% of those it infects. All this means that we can conclude with some confidence that the covid-19 virus began its life in a bat in China and started to spread into people. That is all that is known for absolute certainty about the origins of the virus, almost anyone who claims to know any more is lying. That being said I will now go through some of the conspiracy theories surrounding the origins of the theory to discuss the merits and flaws in each of them.

## The Wuhan Institute of Virology

Of all the theories about the origins of the virus, the most realistic is that it was accidentally released from the Wuhan Institute of Virology. Although again I should stress that we cannot know for certain. The cov-19 virus is most similar genetically to a coronavirus variant known as "RaTG13". This variant has only ever been reported as being found in the Yunnan province of China. In 2012 three miners in Yunnan died of pneumonia they got whilst working in bat infested caves. Blood samples were taken and sent to the Wuhan institute of virology, where that version of the coronavirus (RaTG13) was identified and published. Geographically, Yunnan is a little over 1 500 km away from Wuhan. If the virus originated in the wild and spread to the human population, there are many large cities between the two where the outbreak would have originated from. So we are left with two distinct possibilities. A bat carried the virus 1 500 km from Yunnan to Wuhan without infecting anyone *en route*; or the virus was being studied in the Wuhan institute of Virology and accidentally got exposed and spread to the human population. For me the latter seems the most likely. It is also worth pointing out that this is not a criticism of the Chinese research centres or lab safety in different countries. Before we in the west get all high and mighty about the Chinese letting a virus accidentally escape from a research lab we should really look at our own track record. Smallpox was eradicated from the world in 1977. However, the last death from smallpox was recorded in 1978 when it escaped into an air vent at a research hospital in Birmingham, England.

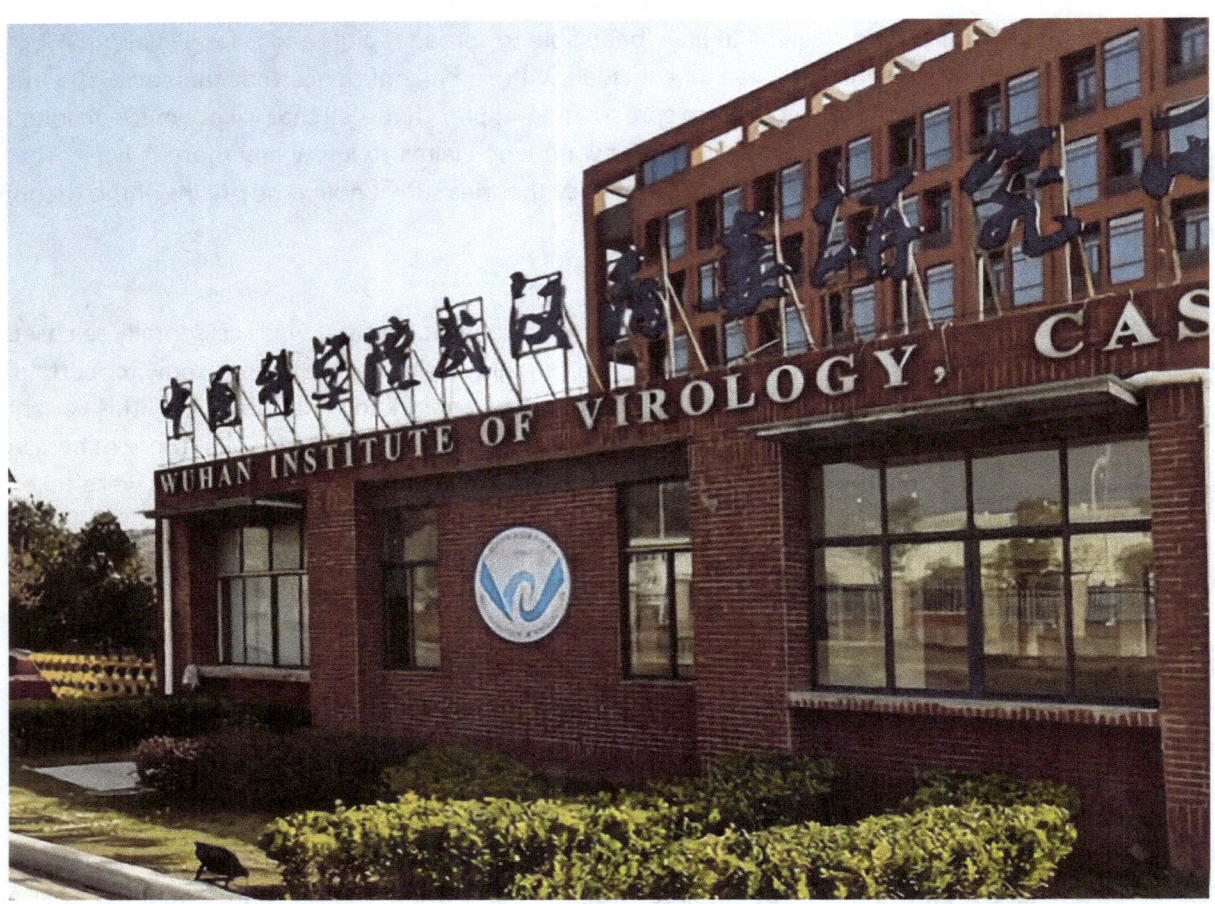

There are those who question why labs like the Wuhan institute of virology exist and what they are doing with the viruses. Accusing the Chinese government of trying to make biological weapons out of the virus. Often conveniently forgetting that just about every country in the world has virology labs that store and study deadly viruses like Ebola and Smallpox. These labs are almost always trying to develop vaccines and treatments for infection. Even if they are trying to turn them into weapons, which some of them are, you would still want an antidote for your own people if you ever released them. This is why I am almost certain that if this virus got out of a lab it was an accident. Why would you release a biological weapon on your own people? Especially before you had a vaccine or treatment. Likewise, most countries are reluctant to stop this research because they believe that their enemies are doing similar research, much like the nuclear arms race. Every nation is trying to develop treatments for their own population in case a foreign enemy releases a virus against them.

It could be asked why this lab was looking at this specific coronavirus? Wouldn´t it be weird if they didn't? After the 2002 SARS-coV outbreak, if a new coronavirus emerged and it turned out the Chinese hadn't even been monitoring coronaviruses or studying them, wouldn't that be a case of extreme negligence? As I said at the start of this section, we may never know the truth about where this virus comes from, but given the geography, the similarity to the RaTG13 strain and the global precedent for viruses escaping from labs; my personal opinion is that an accidental release of the virus at the Wuhan Institute of Virology is the most likely origin story. The only argument against this theory is that between 1-7 million people in china get sick from viruses that jump to them from bats. It is difficult to sequence and study all of these viruses so perhaps the RaTG13 variant is not the most similar variant in reality, but only the most similar coronavirus to cov-19 that we know about. There is a chance that a more similar variant than RaTG13 exists and evolved near Wuhan and has gone undetected for a long time.

## The Huanan seafood wholesale market

A "wet market" in which bats are sold as food was reported as being the epicentre for the covid-19 outbreak. Of the first 41 cases a reported, 27 of those infected worked in or had visited this market in a very short period of time. Before I go into the likelihood of the virus originating in the food market I would like to point out that the market is only 14km from the Wuhan Institute of Virology and if a contagious individual visited the market and infected a seller, there is a chance all these cases were spread by human to human contact, including by someone who worked at the virology institute. If the virus didn't transfer from person to person in the market, did it go from an animal to a person in the market?

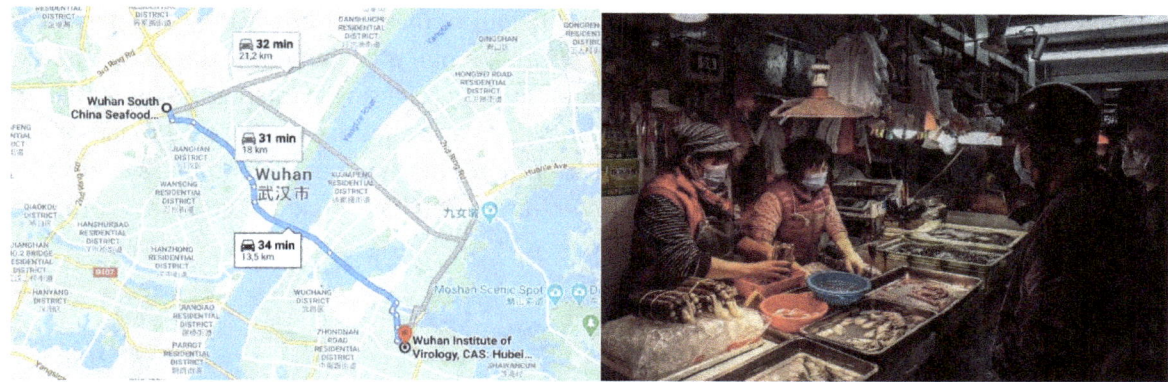

These open air wet markets, which are not dissimilar to farmer's markets in the west, are potential breeding grounds for viruses and it is entirely possible for a virus to jump between species. Ebola and HIV are examples of viruses that have previously jumped from animals to humans. To do so the bodily fluids of an infected animal needs to come into contact with the fluids of the new host species. Given that in these markets there are many different species of animal, all cramped together in confined spaces and the animals are being slaughtered on site, there is a distinct risk that the blood, tears, faeces or pus of an animal could get breathed in by a person in these markets. However, eating food contaminated with the virus would not be a problem if the food was cooked properly. The virus is inactivated by high temperatures and the MERS-coronavirus doesn't spread by eating camel meat that has been properly cooked.

While this theory is definitely plausible, i.e. there is a chance the virus mutated in an animal at the market and then spread to people. The similarity of the covid-19 virus to the RaTG13 strain which was being studied just a 30 min drive away makes that a more probable source of the virus, in my opinion.

## 5G wireless networks

Some conspiracy theories are so farfetched and so devoid of any grounding in reality they are actually very difficult to discuss seriously. This is one of those theories. I have already given an account of what the virus is, so I will now try and explain what 5G wireless networks are. 5G literally stands for the fifth generation of the wireless internet. It has faster download speeds than 4G, which our mobile phones currently use. One of the exciting things about 5G is that it is comparatively as fast as the Wi-Fi in our homes. So in the future you may not need a broadband provider for your home and you mobile, but everything could be done through your 5G network. The way this works is that your device sends and receives radio waves to the nearest cellular tower. Transferring data each way by modulating the frequency of the radio waves. Just like an old FM radio. Virions are too small to contain antennas, transmitters, etc. There is absolutely no connection between the two. The only reason that could possibly explain the genesis of this theory is that most 5G technology is being developed in China, where cov-19 originates; and that the 5G network (new cellular towers) were being rolled out and installed when the virus began to spread. This is a complete coincidence. The two things are in no way related to each other.

## SARS-cov-2 infections

### How the immune system responds to a viral infection

The first biological event that happens within you when a virus enters your body is that your immune system detects that a virus is present. The first line of defence in your immune system are cells known as "macrophages", these are very large cells, by cell standards, which swallow whole any pathogens and digest them using specialist enzymes that can digest (break apart) pretty much anything biological. You have macrophages present and circulating throughout your entire body, they are particularly concentrated in areas where pathogens (bacteria, viruses, fungi, etc.) can enter the body (the skin, eyes, lungs, etc.). Macrophages also trigger "inflammation" by releasing cytokines, Inflammation will be explained in more detail below. Cytokines are small proteins that are released by macrophages, that act as messengers, being transported around the body warning your entire immune system about the infection and getting them to travel to the infect area. You can think of Cytokines as the Paul Revere of the immune system.

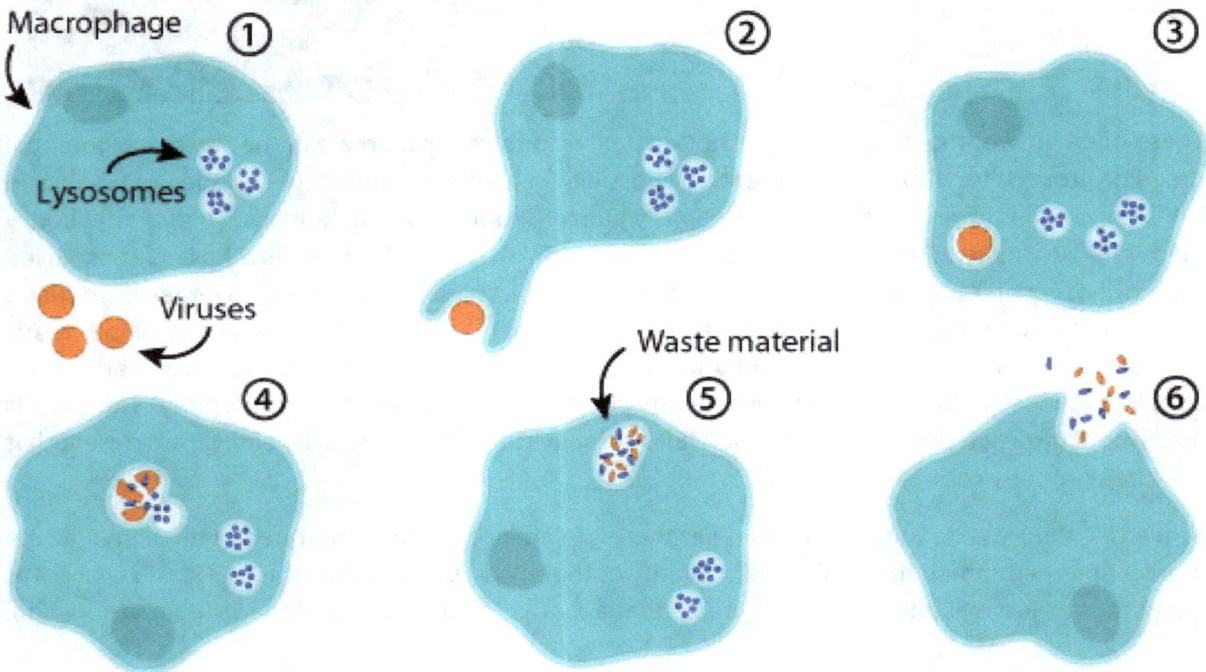

The first type of immune cells that rush to fight off the infection are "neutrophils". These will start to kill anything in the infected area, bacteria, viruses and even your own cells by either "eating them" (the technical term is phagocytosis) just like macrophages or by releasing toxins that kill cells close to them. Neutrophils also build biological barriers around the infected area to stop the disease spreading. For most minor infections, this is usually where the process stops as it is enough to kill off minor infections.

For more serious infections, such as SARS-cov-2, for which the initial immune response is not enough; "antigen presenting cells" become involved to help fight off infections in a more specialised manner. "Antigen" is a technical term to describe the part of an invading species (usually a protein) that your immune system can recognise and bind to. Antigen presenting cells will engulf the virus and break it into smaller pieces, keeping the different component proteins of the virus intact. These antigen presenting cells will then travel to the nearest lymph nodes, small glands spread throughout your body that contain a library of "T-cells" and "B-cells".

T-cells are a type of white blood cell made from stem cells in your bone marrow but are then sent to the thymus gland to mature. It is this process in the thymus (a small organ in your chest, between your heart and throat) that gives the T-cells their name, with the "T" literally referring to the thymus. T-cells have specialised "arms" that can bind to specific proteins that they recognise. When the antigen presenting cells expose proteins from an infection you have had before, T-cells with arms that bind to those specific proteins will recognise them. If you have had an infection before the T-cell will bind to the antigens exposed by the antigen presenting cells and become activated. Once a T-cell becomes activated it starts to duplicate itself. Some of these duplicates become memory T-cells which are stored to fight of future infections, whilst other go to the site of the infection. Every lymph node in your body contains T-cells specific to every infection you have ever had in your life, as well those passed down by your mother in her breast milk. When the killer T-cells arrive at the site of the infection, they look for infected cells and then kill them. All of your cells (except red blood cells) have what are known as "major histocompatibility complexes" (MHCs), which sound more complicated than they really are. These just take proteins from within the cell and expose them to the outside of the cell. If the cell has been infected these MHCs will take the viral proteins being made inside the cell and hold them up outside the cell so that killer T-cells can come along and bind to them. If the cell is not infected the killer t-cells won't do them any harm, but when they do find an infected cell, they release chemicals that kill the cell and therefore stop more virus being made.

As well as T-cells, your immune system has B-cells, so called because they are formed and develop in your bones. B-cells are in some ways very similar to T cells; in that they are stored in your lymphatic system and are activated by cytokines and antigen presenting cells. However, the way that they fight off infection is quite different. The description of T-cells above shows how they can trigger the death of infected host cells to stop your cells from making more copies of the virus. But what about the virions that are not inside these cells but are floating around outside the cells after they have been released? There are T-cells that can, in some cases, stick to and destroy pathogens, but in general we can think of B-cells as being responsible for dealing with the virions outside of cells. B-cells are activated by ingesting (swallowing) the antigens from antigen presenting cells and then developing "antibodies" for them.

You will have no doubt heard about antibodies, they are mentioned constantly in the news, they are important for vaccinations as well as diagnostic tests so are worth understanding in detail. Antibodies are proteins, not enzymes as they do not catalyse any reactions. They are "Y" shaped, see the figure below.

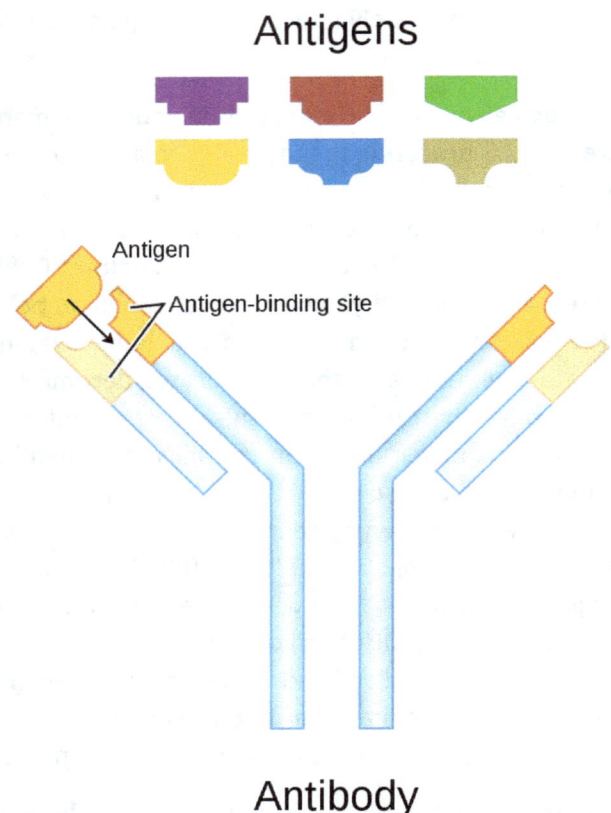

There are various different types of antibody but their basic structure is the same. There is a "conserved region", the blue, bottom part of the image above that is always the same for every antibody of that type. Then there is the "variable" region that binds to the antigen, the yellow top regions in the picture. When your B-cells are fighting an infection they will develop antibodies that stick to the antigen they are shown by the antigen presenting cells. They do this by quickly going through a host of different amino acid sequences within the variable region until they find a sequence that will stick to the protein presented. You have lots of B-cells working simultaneously on the same antigens (in the case of cov-19 the antigen of interest is the spike protein) and quite often they your immune system will produce antibodies with different amino acid sequences that bind to the same antigen. They can do so either by binding to a different part of the antigen or sometimes both sequences will bind to the same spot on the antigen but one sequence will bind better than the other. There is also a chance of variation between people, if two people are infected with the exact same virus, it may be that one person's B-cells found a better amino acid sequence than the others. This is just down to luck, both antibodies have been selected because they stick to the antigen so are still effective. Once your B-cells have found antibodies that stick to the antigen, they begin to mass produce those antibodies and make more B cells with the genetic sequence for these antibodies. The antibodies are then released and bind to the antigen of the virions lying around outside of cells. Once they have bound to the virion, different types of antibody do different things. Remember that the yellow, top of the Y shape has bound to the spike proteins and the bottom blue part of the antibody in the picture is pointing away from the virion.

This is where the different types of antibody become important. Some antibodies are designed to just stick to the spike proteins of viruses, by doing this so they physically block the spike proteins from being able to stick to ACE2 receptors, preventing them from infecting any host cells. The Y-shape of antibodies means that they can stick to two virions, one through each variable arm. By doing so they can form clusters of the virus, herding them together to make it easier for macrophages to eat them, effectively gathering up lots of crumbs and sticking them together for the macrophages to eat. Other antibodies have conserved regions that, once the antibody has bound to the antigen, will activate killer T-cells and neutrophils to come along and eat or poison the pathogen.

B-cells, like T-cells, can do one of two things after developing antibodies, they can either become "killer B-cells" which go to the site of the infection and produce lots of antibodies, or they can become memory B-cells, which live in your lymphatic system and will store the code for your antibodies for future. If your body gets infected by the same virus again; these memory B-cells will be triggered by antigen presenting cells and can quickly mass produce antibodies to fight off the infection. Interestingly you get antibodies not just through your immune system learning from your own previous infections, but antibodies cross the placenta from the mother to the baby, so we are all born with generations of inherited antibodies. It is a common misconception that if you have antibodies you cannot get the same infection again. You absolutely can. Only when you have antibodies your body has been trained in how to deal with that specific pathogen and can quickly mobilise a specific response to deal with it. This means that you won´t normally get as sick and will be able to get better quicker. Antibodies are discussed further in the sections on Antibody diagnostics and vaccines in this book.

That is the generalised method by which your immune system will respond to a general invasion. In truth there are people who devote their entire lives to studying just one or two of each of these types of cells or even just a couple of the proteins within them and what they do, so it is not easy to get your head around. I realise there are is a lot of jargon in there so if have become lost or confused please do not worry. Your immune system is a complicated and marvellous thing, I have tried to summarise all of the above into a single, simpler to understand paragraph:

When a virus enters your body, macrophages (large, hungry proteins); will come along and eat them. These macrophages will make and release cytokines, the biological Paul Revere´s that run around telling the entire immune system that something is wrong. Neutrophils will then turn up and start to release poisons within the area to kill anything and everything that might compromise the safety of all the healthier, further away, cells. Specialist antigen presenting cells will then come in if this is not enough, grab the invader and split it up into its constituent parts. It will then go to your immune library to find B-cells and T-cells that recognise any of the individual parts of the pathogen. If the infection is recognised in your library, then these cells will kick into action and start to replicate and mass produce themselves and antibodies to quickly fight off the infection. If this is a new infection, your body needs to train and develop B-cells and T-cells to recognise and fight this antigen. Once this is done the T-cells will find infected host cells and tell them to kill themselves, stopping you from making any more copies of the virus, and the B-cells will start making antibodies that stick to the virus and prevent them infecting new cells and allow other cells to start clearing them out of your body.

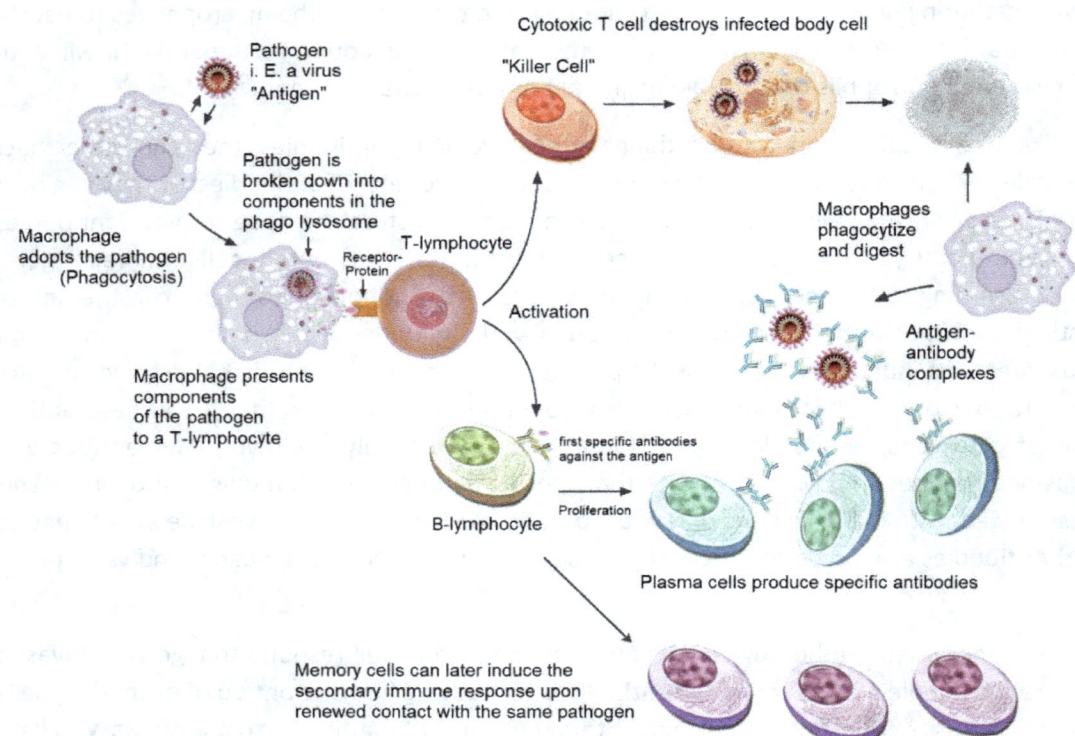

# SARS-nCoV-2019 Symptoms and how to manage them

One of the most surprising and confusing aspects of this virus is the broad spectrum of different symptoms that those infected present. Some people are completely asymptomatic (have absolutely no symptoms and feel completely healthy) whilst others get such severe pneumonia that it eventually leads to their death. In most cases, those who do get sick with covid-19 will have some but not all of the symptoms listed below and which ones they get differ from person to person.

I will start off by listing all of the reported symptoms before going through them all one by one in more detail to explain what is causing them on a physiological level. I have also included practical tips of ways of alleviating any of the symptoms if you get any of them.

Common coronavirus symptoms:

- Fever
- Dry cough
- Tiredness

Less common symptoms:

- Aches and pains
- Diarrhoea
- Conjunctivitis (inflammation or infection of the eye)
- Headache
- Loss of taste
- Loss of smell
- Skin rash (discoloured fingers or toes)

Rarer, serious symptoms:

- Difficulty breathing
- Pneumonia
- Chest pain or pressure
- Paralysis

It may surprise you to learn that the virus itself does not really cause any of these symptoms. In fact, all of your symptoms are as a result of your immune system trying to fight off the infection. This is perhaps one reason why there is so much variation in symptoms between different people, their immune systems are all different so react differently to the virus.

## Inflammation

Before going through the different symptoms, there is a common thread that will arise in almost all of them. Most of the symptoms are caused by inflammation, but what exactly is inflammation? Inflammation is again a product of your immune system fighting off an infection. The exact biological processes are quite complicated and you could spend years studying all of the biological pathways that lead to inflammation. In short though, it is triggered by cytokines, those Paul Revere type proteins mentioned above, which are released by macrophages and neutrophils, the first responders of the immune system that non-specifically attack the infection.

Inflammation can be caused by anything that could be perceived as harmful to the body. Physically inflammation is: swelling, heat, redness, pain and loss of function in an area of the body. The main purpose of inflammation is to fight off any infection. The rush of immune cells and build-up of dead cells in a confined area inevitably causes it to swell (also a result of increased blood flow and water to the area). The heat is caused by localised increases in temperature to help kill infected cells and pathogens. The pain, redness and loss of function are also as a result of increased blood flow and temperatures and swelling. Once your immune cells have digested the infected cells or virions, they kill themselves and end up becoming puss. Puss is simply your own dead immune cells that have "eaten" and destroyed as many viruses as possible before killing themselves.

The most common anti-inflammatory drug is ibuprofen. In March of 2020 the French authorities recommended that those with covid-19 symptoms should not use ibuprofen as it led to more severe symptoms in those infected with covid-19. The theory was that taking Ibuprofen made your cells produce more ACE2 receptors, increasing the likelihood of the virus binding to one and infecting it. However, this was found to be based on purely anecdotal evidence and was not supported by any scientific findings. Most governments have now withdrawn their advice against using ibuprofen and believe it is safe to do so after proper scientific studies. Interestingly there was an 80% decrease in Ibuprofen sales in France immediately after the announcement. With that being said you should always consult with your doctor before taking any medication if you have SARS-cov-2, if your symptoms are not severe the inflammation will help your immune system fight off the virus, but if it is too severe it can have serious health consequences.

## Fever

When your body detects that there is an infection your immune system kicks in and starts to fight it off. There are many ways by which it does this, one of which is to increase your body temperature. Most pathogens (the technical term for all the viruses, bacteria, etc. that can infect you and make you sick) have evolved to be very effective at the normal human body temperature. By raising your temperature, your immune system can inactivate (kill without breaking apart) many pathogens. This is a pretty crude method of fighting off infections as it can also cause harm to your own body cells but is just one of the ways we have evolved to fight off dangerous diseases. So what is a normal body temperature? A healthy body temperature is 37 °C (98.6 F) and is very finely controlled by your body. Anything higher than this is considered a fever. If your body temperature goes above 40 °C (104 F) then you begin to suffer from "heat stroke". Heat stroke is often confused with heat exhaustion. Heat exhaustion is what you feel if you have been sitting out in the sun or next to a heat source for too long and feel uncomfortable or sick. Sitting in a cooler environment and drinking water can cure heat exhaustion. Heat stroke on the other hand is a very serious medical condition where your internal body temperature rises above 40 °C (104 F), it is comparable in seriousness to having a heart attack and anyone who has a temperature above 40 °C (104 F) should seek immediate medical attention and will need to be hospitalised, usually for several weeks. There have been incidences reported of people suffering from SARS-cov-2 who have developed heat stroke as a result of their high fevers. If you have SARS-cov-2 it is recommended that you use a thermometer to record your temperature several times a day to make sure you don´t overheat. Another effect of raising your body temperature is what is known as "vasodilation", the expansion of your blood vessels, this happens particularly in infected areas and is triggered by the immune system to increase blood flow to the area. The result of this is that your immune cells can get better access to the infected areas as well as flooding the area with nutrients that your cells need to fight off an infection.

- **TIPS:**
  If you or someone you know has SARS-cov-2 and develops a high fever, it is important to drink plenty of fluids. They will most likely be sweating a lot. It is important to remember that when you sweat you lose a lot of salts as well as water, if your salts get too low you will feel tired and weak. Drinking isotonic sports drinks will replenish your salts as well as fluids.
- Excessive sweating will make you feel uncomfortable, regular showering or bathing will not only make you feel fresher but can lower your body temperature if you overheat. Not to mention smell better, which if you lose your sense of smell you may not notice.
- Paracetamol also works to lower your body temperature but should be used sparingly, always consult with your doctor before taking paracetamol to reduce your fever as taking too much can make things worse.

## Dry cough

When a cough is "dry", that means that you are not coughing up any phlegm. This is often caused by an irritation in your throat, often a tickling sensation can be felt. This can partly be put down to dehydration, usually as a result of increased sweating due to a fever. However, the main cause is inflammation of the lungs and throat.

**TIPS:**

- Drinking tea with honey is good for soothing a sore throat.
- In some cultures, including my own, there is an old wives' tale that drinking a warm whisky or other spirit is good for a sore throat. Whilst alcohol is an anaesthetic and might reduce the pain, dealing with alcohol puts a burden on you liver and takes valuable resources away from fighting the infection so this is not recommended.
- There are various over the counter lozenges and cough sweets that can alleviate the pain of a dry cough.
- It is important to practice good cough etiquette by coughing into the inside of your elbow to avoid spreading the disease
- If you are coughing and have SARS-cov-2 you are spreading the virus. You have a responsibility to self-isolate until you get a negative PCR test. If you fail to do so you may be responsible for someone else getting infected and possibly dying.

## Tiredness

Feeling lethargic is common for most infections. As your immune system is fighting off diseases it needs lots more energy to do so. This causes a drain on your bodies energy reserves and makes you feel tired. When you are asleep your heart rate and other bodily functions slow down allowing your body to devote more of its energy to fighting the infection and repairing any damage to the body caused in the process.

From personal experience of having had SARS-cov-2 in November of 2020, I can testify that the tiredness was one of the most "severe" symptoms. I am a fit and healthy man in my early thirties, going on 10 km runs 3-4 times a week. When healthy I will sleep for 6-8 hours per night and wake up feeling refreshed. When I had corona, I would sleep 14-16 hours a day and nap during the time I was awake. Just getting up the energy to go and shower or wash the dishes was difficult. This is a personal experience however and varies from person to person.

**TIPS:**

- Tiredness is your body´s way of telling you to take a rest. Go with it and get as much sleep as you can, it is good for you.
- Family members and friends can get stressed if they know you have an infection and don't hear from you. Please be considerate when someone has SARS-cov-2, they need their sleep and peace. Personally having had 5-10 people insisting on calling three times a day each to check on my progress was actually quite tiring and stressful. I don't want to sound ungrateful and am very touched that those people care about my wellbeing, but please be considerate of those who are sick, they do need to time and space to just sleep and recover. Perhaps arrange to post on social media or in a group chat on a regular basis to let everyone know how you are getting on.

### Less common symptoms

### Aches and pains

These can vary from mild to severe and show up in different parts of the body. Personally when I had SARS-cov-2, I had very bad aches and pains in my lower back and my thighs. These are caused by inflammation in those areas, which may be as a result of the virus accumulating in those areas. Alternatively, it could be that the inflammatory cytokines have accumulated in those areas without the virus. In order to lessen these aches and pains the virus or inflammatory need to be flushed out of the area.

**TIPS:**

- Massaging the affected muscles can increase blood flow and try to spread any virus or cytokines from the area which will reduce the inflammation.
- Applying something cold like an ice pack can lower the temperature locally and reduce inflammation.
- Again, showering can help cool the area.
- Anti-inflammatory drugs can help but should only be used in severe cases and always after consulting with your doctor.

### Diarrhoea

The cells in your intestines, like your lungs, have a lot of ACE2 receptors so the virus can spread to and infect these cells. The resulting inflammation can lead not only to Diarrhoea but also a loss of appetite, stomach pains and vomiting.

**TIPS:**

- One of the main things to watch out for with Diarrhoea is dehydration. It is important to keep drinking energy drinks rich in salts to replenish fluids and salts.
- Before taking any medication to combat Diarrhoea you should consult your doctor. Depending on the medication you take it could make things much worse. Stronger antidiarrhoeatics (drugs that stop diarrhoea), are known to prolong other types of gut infection so may make

you more sick. This happens because these drugs stop your normal gut movements, which means your body can not get rid of the viral ad cell waste. In other words, your body is trying to get rid of waste that is contaminated and you are preventing it from doing so. It is therefore not advisable to take any medication unless your doctor thinks your diarrhoea is so severe it is causing more harm than the virus.

## Conjunctivitis

Commonly called "pinkeye", conjunctivitis is any sort of inflammation in the conjunctiva (a small membrane that covers your eyes and the inside of your eyelids). This is typically caused by the virus spreading to and infecting the cells that make up this membrane. It will normally clear up on its own within a week or two.

**TIPS:**

- Try applying a cold damp cloth over the eyes to lessen inflammation.
- Over the counter eye drops are safe to use.
- Never wear contact lenses if you have any form of eye infection or irritation.

## Headaches

The types of headaches that you get from a covid-19 infection feel like a constant high pressure throughout the entire head. These are distinctly different from migraines which are a throbbing pain throughout the head with a sensitivity to light and/or sound. There are two methods by which a covid-19 infection may be causing these headaches. The first is again due to cytokines causing inflammation, the blood vessels within your brain start to swell and cause an increase of pressure within the head. These types of headache will usually subside when the infection has been dealt with.

The second more worrying headaches the virus causes are less well understood and potentially more dangerous. There are some SARS-cov-2 survivors who have reported having these headaches for several months after the infection. Current thinking on this is that the virus has gotten into the brain and infected brain cells. If you continue to have headaches or feel a pressure in your head after the infection has subsided, you should speak about this with your doctor.

**TIPS:**

- Plenty of sleep and water are universal cures for everything.
- Over the counter headache pills can also be used quite safely.
- Stress can contribute to making headaches worse, taking a break from social media and the news can alleviate headaches.

## Loss of taste (Ageusia) and smell (Anosmia)

I have decided to deal with these together as our taste and smell are closely linked. A loss of smell will impair our sense of taste, as smell is an important part of eating. These have come to be almost defining symptoms of the covid-19 pandemic, even inspiring corona challenges on social media where people smell and eat horrible things because they cannot taste. But this is actually quite a common side effect of most viral infections.

The exact method of how this happens biologically is not known. What we do know is that smell and taste nerve cells have no ACE2 receptors so are not themselves infected and killed. The current best explanation, which has not been proven, is that the cells near your nerve cells get infected and swollen and this squeezing of the nerve cells stops them working. Hopefully with more time the truth will be found out. The sense of smell and taste will almost always return, for some people this takes longer due to the amount of damage done that needs to be repaired. Usually this is recovered with days or weeks but it has been reported to take months. Whether the damage can be permanent is impossible to say as SARS-cov-2 is so new.

**TIPS:**

- There is nothing medically that can be done to reverse or lessen this.
- Smelling vinegar is a good test of how much smell you still have, try smelling vinegar several times a day to see if your smell is coming back yet.
- If you cannot taste or smell, perhaps this is a good time to embrace that and start eating healthier foods you may not normally like. Also, there is no point eating junk food if you cannot taste it. Make the best of a bad situation and eat a healthy diet, it will help you get better quicker as well.

## Skin rash

It took quite a while before skin rashes were identified as a symptom of covid-19 infections. The main reason for this is that there are so many different types of rash that corona can cause and they vary from person to person and come at different stages of the infection. Rashes are caused by inflammation or the virus infecting skin cells. The type of rash that usually develops earliest is a "urticarial" type of rash (commonly called hives). These are rashes where you have raised pale red or skin coloured bumps of plaques. These are usually very itchy. They can appear anywhere on the body including the face and mouth where they cause the lips to swell. If the mouth swells to the point where breathing is difficult seek immediate medical attention. Normally these rashes will come and go over several hours. These are directly caused by histamine (a chemical responsible for inflammation) at the skin and can be treated by anti-histamines.

Erythemato-papular or erythemato-vesicular rashes are red bumpy (chicken-pox like) rashes that are also very itchy and can appear anywhere on the body, but tend to be found more on the elbows, knees, hands and feet. Occasionally they will have a warm heat to them but this is not always the case. These rashes are longer lasting and can take weeks to fully heal. They form much later on in the disease progression with some cases being reported several weeks after the patient has recovered from the virus. Personally I developed rashes like this on my feet a full three months after recovering from SARS-cov-2.

Chilblains used to be a rash people got from having poor circulation to their hands and feet. Usually in the winter when spending time in the cold. Characterised by a redness or purple discolouration of the skin and some swelling of the area, typically the hands or feet. For some reason in corona this tends to affect the young more than the elderly and is onset later in, or even weeks after, the infection. These rashes are not typically itchy but the swelling can be painful.

## Hives

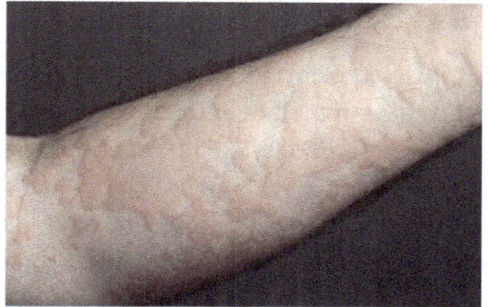

## Hives on the mouth

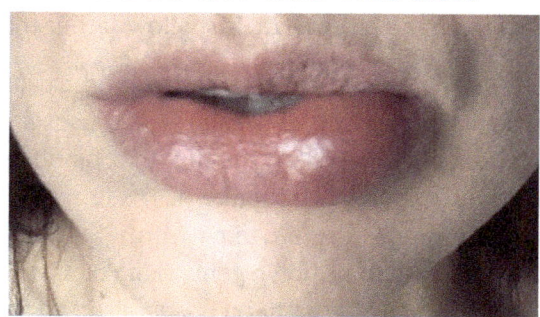

## Erythemato-papular rashes

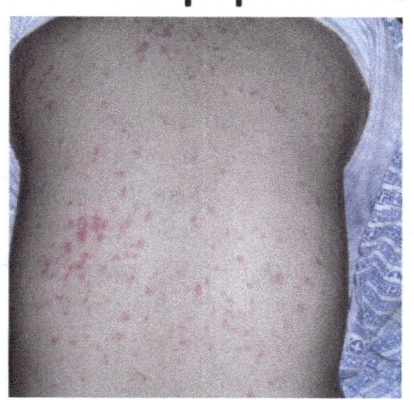

## Chilblains

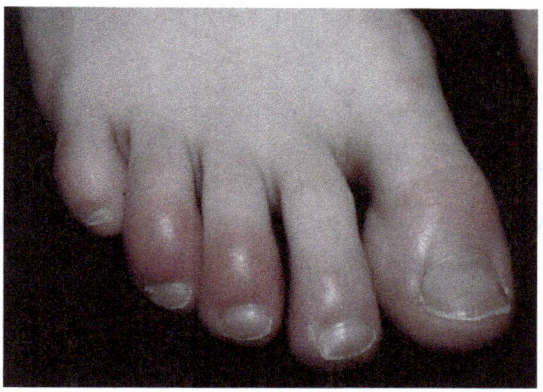

**TIPS:**

- Avoid itching the rashes as you can open the skin which will possibly get infected and can lead to scarring.
- Apply corticosteroids or take an oatmeal bath to make the rashes less itchy.
- To avoid scratching in your sleep try sleeping with gloves or socks over your hands or the rash.
- Applying a cold compress will help reduce the temperature and swelling and make the rash less itchy.
- Your doctor may prescribe antihistamines to help treat a rash.

# Rarer symptoms

Before continuing I should point out that the rarer conditions listed here are also the most serious and can be fatal. Anyone experiencing these symptoms should already be hospitalised or seek medical attention. There are no "tips" on how to alleviate these symptoms as they require treatment by trained medical professionals.

## Difficulty breathing

The difficulty in breathing arises from the damage caused to the lungs by the virus spreading, infecting and killing lung cells; as well as the damage that the immune response does to the lungs while trying to fight off the infection. Lungs work by having a very large surface area over which they expose blood to the air; oxygen then binds to blood cells and carbon dioxide is released. As more and more of the lung cells are destroyed, the surface area of the lungs decreases and less oxygen can get into your blood. Another way of explaining this is that as the virus spreads through the lungs they effectively get smaller. A normal breath will not bring as much oxygen into the blood as it used to before the infection. In mild to moderate infections this will manifest itself as difficulty breathing, or just a general feeling that every breath is shallow rather than deep.

The accepted method of testing blood oxygen levels is to use an oximeter, a small electronic device that fits on the end of the finger and uses a pulsing light to determine the amount of oxygen in your blood. This is based on the fact that blood will absorb different amounts of light depending on how much oxygen it has bound to it. These are relatively cheap devices that can be bought online. Normal healthy ranges are anything from 95-100 % oxygen saturation. Different countries have different recommendations but in general, if you have one of these devices and your blood oxygen drops below 90-92% you will need to be hospitalised and treated with oxygen enriched air. You should however be careful when using oximeters as the values they give can vary when standing, sitting, and on different fingers. The best results are obtained from the middle finger of your right hand whilst sitting in an upright position.

The initial treatment for more severe cases is to give someone oxygen enriched air. Normal air contains about 21% oxygen. By giving someone a supply of artificial air with a higher oxygen concentration, the parts of the lungs that are still healthy will be able to take in enough oxygen to compensate for the damaged lung tissue. In the most severe cases the lungs are not able to function properly by themselves and the patient needs to be put on a ventilator. Ventilators are machines that mechanically expand and collapse the lungs, filling them with oxygen enriched air and removing the carbon dioxide breathed out. These are only used in the most severe cases where the lungs are so badly damaged that they are incapable of doing this work themselves.

Difficulty in breathing is also a side effect of pneumonia.

## Pneumonia

The technical definition of pneumonia is an inflammation in the air sacs of the lungs caused by an infection, usually resulting in pus or liquid filling the lungs. As stated earlier, the lungs need to have a very large surface area to get enough oxygen to transfer between the blood and the air. In order to do this, your lungs have evolved to have a lot of tubes and small sacs that fill with air when you breathe in. These look a lot like bunches of grapes hanging off of branches, with the air running inside the stalks and filling the grapes.

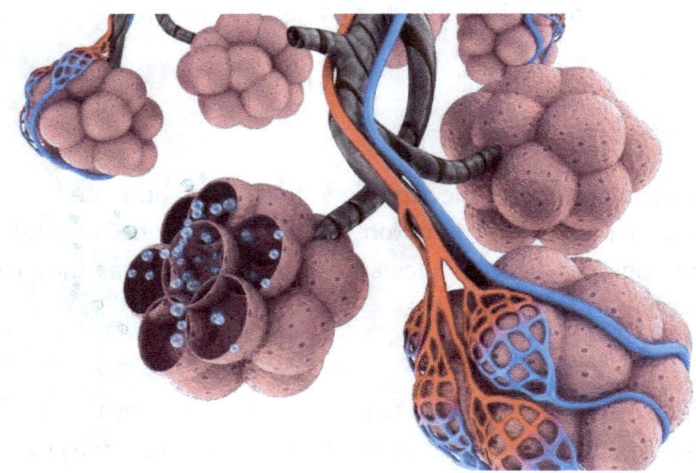

When someone has pneumonia, the immune system fights off the invading pathogen as well as infected cells. In the case of airborne pathogens, the infected cells are those that are directly exposed to the air. As mentioned earlier, pus is formed by immune cells eating viruses and infected cells. So there is a build-up of puss as well as fluids (usually water which gathers in the area due to inflammation) inside the air sacs. As the pus and fluids build up they block the transfer of oxygen from the air into the blood and carbon dioxide going the other way, in effect drowning the patient. News reports from the frontline of SARS-Cov-2 treatment usually show patients being routinely being flipped in their beds (a procedure called "proning"). This is to try and get the fluids that are building in the air sacs to flow into one half of the lungs and free up the other half for better breathing. Since the fluids/pus is being produced constantly throughout the lungs the patients need to be flipped at regular intervals from their back to their sides and their stomach's in turn.

## Chest pain or pressure

Chest pain can be a result of inflammation and damage of lung tissue or pneumonia. There are no reported cases of anyone having chest pain without other SARS-coV-2 symptoms. If you are experiencing chest pain but no other symptoms you probably do not have corona but there is no harm in being tested. There have been several studies showing an increase in people suffering chest pains due to what is being dubbed "corona anxiety". What seems like a constant influx of bad news and fear from the media, worries about job security and having to self-isolate is not good for people's mental health and has caused increases in anxiety, which can cause chest pains. The genuine scientific advice is to try and reduce your exposure to news reports and social media if you are feeling overwhelmed and anxious about the situation. It is also helpful to know that you are not alone, everyone is in the same position and going through the same emotions.

## Paralysis

This is perhaps the rarest of the symptoms and even in severe and fatal cases is quite rare. SARS-cov-2 induced paralysis is caused by "Guillain-Barré syndrome". In such cases the immune system mistakenly thinks that nerve cells are dangerous and starts to kill them. This leads to muscle weakness and eventually paralysis. There have only been a handful of SARS-cov-2 cases where paralysis has been observed.

## Other symptoms

One thing that should be borne in mind is that this is a new virus and new symptoms are constantly being identified. It took quite a while for people to identify that this virus, which normally infects the lungs, could spread to the brain. Other symptoms are not just neurological, there is also evidence that the virus can increase blood clotting (forming scabs); which can lead to strokes, heart disease and heart attacks. The problem scientist have is trying to mine through all the data available that is coming so quickly and trying to exclude some symptoms that may be a result of complications with other underlying health conditions. It is entirely possible that before long more symptoms will be added to this list and some may be taken off.

One very strange symptom that merits some discussion is that of reports of lung scarring in asymptomatic patients. People who test positive for corona but have no symptoms will quite naturally think that they have gotten quite lucky. However, imaging of their lungs show that there is significant damage in about half of asymptomatic positive cases. It is not known whether these images are just of unhealthy lungs that will heal with time, or signs of scarring within the lungs that can have long term health implications, only time will tell. There is much that we still need to learn about this pandemic but one of the most interesting questions is how people who have damaged lungs were completely asymptomatic. Logically you would think that if people have damaged lung tissue they would show at least some symptoms. The amount of scarring in some of these images is pretty severe. You would expect people to have some difficulty breathing or chest pain when a third of their lungs are scarred or damaged but they are reported as feeling completely fine.

## Long corona

Usually people who have recovered from covid-19 infections will feel better and produce negative PCR test results a few weeks after the first symptoms appear. However, even several weeks and months after the infection there are reports of several symptoms in survivors. It is not possible to say if these will go away or last longer as the pandemic has not been around that long. The persistent symptoms of corona that have so far been identified are:

- Tiredness
- Difficulty breathing
- Problems with memory
- Difficulty concentrating
- Insomnia
- Heart palpitations (irregular heartbeats)
- Dizziness
- Pins and needles
- Joint and muscle pain
- Diarrhoea
- Stomach pains
- Loss of appetite
- Ear aches
- Feeling sick
- Depression
- Anxiety
- Rashes
- Fever
- Cough
- Headaches
- Sore throat
- Loss of smell and/or taste

Some of these can be the result of it taking time for the body to heal and replace the cells destroyed by the virus or the immune response. Some, like depression and anxiety, may be the result of other factors with these being more prevalent in society in general during the pandemic than they were before. But the long term effects of a cov-19 infection are not fully explained or understood and will take more time to understand.

Some viruses are known to "hide" in the body and when released can cause a second bout of an infection or even infect others. The most common places for viruses to hide are the eye, the testes and the brain. That is because these organs are partially shielded from the immune system, because the immune response can cause permanent serious damage to these regions. It is not known if the covid-19 virus is hiding in these organs but if it was that could explain the existence of long corona and how the virus keeps re-emerging after lockdowns.

## How does the coronavirus spread?

As discussed above, the coronavirus infects cells with ACE2 receptors. These are overly abundant in the lungs which is makes the lungs the main route of infection for the virus into the body. The coronavirus can enter the lungs by breathing in air with covid-19 virions suspended in it. Likewise, if the virus lands on a surface that you touch and then you touch your face or eat with your hands without washing them, it is easy to see how it can end up in your mouth or nose and be breathed into your lungs from there. It is important to bear in mind just how small the virions are. At only 50-200 nm in diameter they are extremely small and light; a virion may take a lot longer than you would expect to fall to the ground. However, individual virions aren't exactly released into the air by themselves. Whenever you breathe, sing, whistle, cough, sneeze, speak or yawn, you are releasing "respiratory droplets" into the air. Respiratory droplets are mainly comprised of water and mucus as well as any bacteria or viruses that are present within your lungs, throat, mouth or nose. You can sometimes see the larger droplets of these which fall to the ground within a few seconds, however, there are microscopically small respiratory droplets there as well. These have the same ingredients as the larger droplets but can remain airborne for hours. They can be transported through the environment by wind and drafts. Many countries have imposed social distancing rules which encourage people to keep 1.5 or 2 meters away from each other. Even if you adhere to these rules, if you are in a small room with someone who is corona positive there is a good chance you will breath in the virus. This is one of several reasons that despite these social distancing measures the virus continues to spread throughout the world at an alarming rate.

Once the virus has left the body, how long can it "survive" on a surface and infect others? This is quite a difficult question to answer and depends on a lot more factors than you would initially think. The media has been flooded with reports that the virus can live on say petrol pumps for two weeks, or that it is only viable for a few hours or a couple of days. The numbers differ depending on which report you read. The truth is that it really depends on the surface on which they land and what else has been coughed up or breathed out with the virus. Some surfaces, such as copper, are known to have antibacterial properties and there are some initial reports that the virus will become inactive after only two hours on copper, significantly shorter than stainless steel. We need to be very careful in this discussion to refer to making the virus "unviable". Since viruses are not technically alive and when they land on surfaces that are not friendly to them they are not "killed" and do not "die". The viability of a virus is measured by taking the virus off the surface and seeing if it is still capable of infecting host cells. A lot of surfaces are tested by placing viruses grown in a lab on test surfaces, taking them off and seeing if they are still viable after having been on the surface for different lengths of time. These tests are not necessarily that reliable though. In the real world the virus will land on a surface with mucus, water and everything else breathed out with it, which will change from person to person and day to day. Some of these will help to keep the virus viable for longer and some will inactivate them quicker. Because tests are done under different conditions, with and without mucus from different sources and on different surfaces, there are all sorts of different numbers being thrown around about the viability of virions in the environment. Unfortunately, that means the only appropriate response is to assume the worst, which is that the virus can survive in the environment for several weeks (the longest times reported), or until a surface is cleaned.

## How can we stop the spread of the virus?

### Masks

In order to stop the virus spreading through the air, the only real solution at the moment is to have everyone wear masks. This follows some pretty simple logic, if the virus spreads through breathing you wear something over your mouth and nose to prevent the virus either getting in or out of the two body parts you breathe through (the nose and the mouth). Yet the utter confusion and political ineptitude that has arisen surrounding the use of masks is absolutely staggering. Before I go into how masks work and the difference between different types of masks I would like to point out something that should be obvious to everyone. In 2018, if you went in for an operation in any hospital in the world, you would probably be operated on by surgeon who would be wearing a mask. Masks do not suffocate those who wear them, there are no long or short term health risks from wearing masks unless you are allergic to what they are made out of. It´s not as if surgeons have been suffocating or passing out during surgery for the last hundred years due to excessive mask wearing. If you are allergic, hypoallergenic masks are available. There is no excuse or reason to not wear a mask.

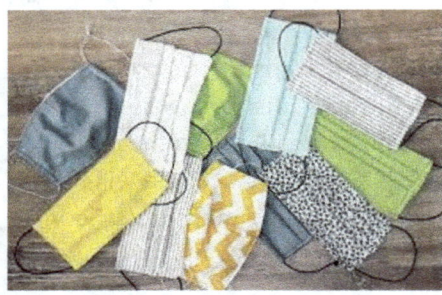 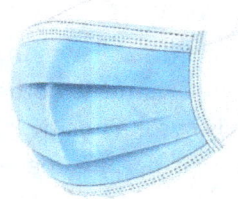 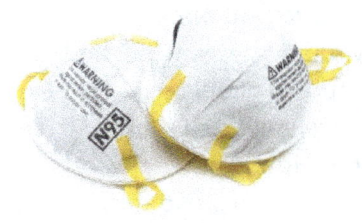

There are a wide variety of masks on the market, from surgical masks to homemade cloth masks and the now famous N95 masks. All these masks work the same way to prevent the virus spreading except the N95 masks which are a special case. Most masks are made from a textile material (usually polypropylene) which is porous so that you can breathe through it. These pores are small enough to physically prevent things like bacteria and human cells that you breathe from passing through them. These pores are usually around 1 000 nm (0.001 mm) in diameter, far bigger than the coronavirus which is around 200 nm in diameter. For some people, that is where the conversation ends and they assume that this means the virions can pass through the masks and they do not keep you safe. However, this completely misunderstands how masks actually work. As mentioned above, when we breath out we breathe respiratory droplets which contain mucus, water, bacteria, human cells, etc. the water in your breath condenses on the inside of a mask when you wear it, next time you wear a mask and take it off just feel how wet the inside of it is. This forms a protective layer of water and mucus that will catch the virus if you breathe it out. However, these masks offer no protection against the virus in the air that you breathe in. Hence you will often hear people saying that masks only work if everyone wears them. If everyone who had the virus wore masks out in public the viral spread would be reduced. This method works with any fabric that gets wet when you wear it in a mask, such as tissues and paper towels. But again this requires that everyone wear a mask. In countries like Sweden where masks are not compulsory the virus is spreading at an alarming rate and those who do wear masks, thinking they are protecting themselves are put in danger by those who choose not to wear masks.

Alternatively, there are N95 masks, these have pores that are on average 95 nm in diameter (hence the name). These will protect the wearer as the air they breathe in will physically filter out anything larger than 95 nm from the air being breathed in, including the 200 nm diameter coronavirus. However, I do not want to get people panicked and rushing to go out and buy N95 masks. Other masks, even homemade ones, will work perfectly well if everyone uses them and uses them properly. There is, at the time of writing, a global shortage on surgical and N95 masks and frontline healthcare workers cannot get hold of them. In my personal opinion, N95 masks should not be sold to the general population, but rather restricted for use by frontline healthcare workers, who are coming into contact with the virus on a daily basis, and the general population should all be made to wear masks in public. At least until N95 mask production can be increased to meet the new global demand.

With that said, masks can be uncomfortable and there are countless people using them wrong, so I have compiled a list of hints and tips on how to wear them properly and make them more comfortable whilst staying safe.

- If you have a homemade mask, change the internal filter (usually a tissue) on a regular basis and wash the masks themselves regularly as well. Regularly means at least once a day. I would recommend to put on a clean mask when leaving the house and not take it off until you come home and clean it or bin it straight away.
- Disposable masks should be disposed of after every public use.
- If the mask is chaffing at the back of your ears you can use the "paperclip trick" to fasten them behind your head, see picture below. You can make a paperclip chain if this is uncomfortably tight.
- The mask should cover both your mouth and nose! It is staggering to see people walking around with the mask over their mouth but not their nose. You can get infected by breathing through both so must cover and protect both the mouth and nose.
- Masks have a metal strip that can be bent and fit over your nose, so this side should be at the top. Bending this strip into a sharp bend in the middle before putting on the mask will make it fit better.
- If the masks are too big, you can twist the ear loops over themselves to tighten the mask.
- If your glasses are steaming up when you wear a mask, it is not properly fitted to your face and needs to be tightened. The top of the mask should lie flush against the face, try tightening using the paperclip trick or twisting the ear loops. Alternatively try taping the top of the mask to your nose using a band aid or breathable adhesive tape. This can also stop the mask slipping down your face.

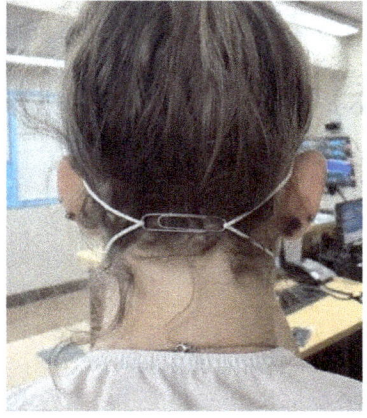
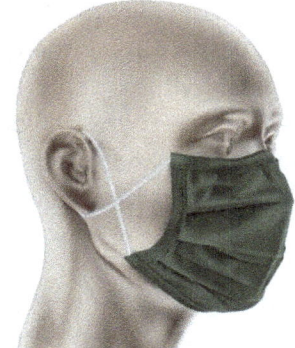

IF MASK IS TOO BIG, ADJUST BY TWISTING AND MAKING A LOOP BEHIND THE EAR FOR A SNUG FIT.

### Washing hands with soap or hand sanitizer

Another method of fighting the spread of the virus is to wash our hands regularly with soap or hand sanitizer. This works by not only killing any virus that you might get on your hands from touching surfaces with the virus on them, but also stops you from then spreading the virus to other surfaces that you touch if you are infected. Both soap and the ethanol in the hand sanitizer are very effective at destroying the virus. I use the word "destroy" rather than "inactivate" for a very good reason. Soap is a "surfactant" it contains lots of molecules that are similar to the lip bilayer in the virus. They chemically break this layer apart and dissolve it, rapidly destroying the viral envelope within a few seconds. The ethanol in hand sanitizer works by a slightly different method but still destroys the virions. When a virion is surrounded by ethanol, it still has water inside its envelope. The water inside the virion starts to rapidly diffuse out of the envelope, causing the virion to burst. The concentration of ethanol at which this process works best is about 70% ethanol but higher concentrations also work.

If you have heard rumours that vodka or other strong spirits kill the virus, well, yes... They do, but they are not as effective at killing the virus as soap or hand sanitizer, which will do so in seconds. Also, it's a bit of a shame to waste your good drink on washing your hands. I also want to make it clear that I don't want a repeat of the infamous "disinfectant incident". Drinking alcohol goes into your stomach, not your lungs so won't cure you. Likewise breathing in ethanol will not kill the virus in your lungs. Once you are infected the virus is inside your cells so drinking or breathing in the vapours of soap, disinfectant or ethanol will just poison you and make things a lot worse. It will not cure your infection. In fact, it is advisable not to drink at all when you have an infection of any sort as it just puts more strain on your liver, where alcohol is broken down.

As well as causing the degradation of the virions, soap and ethanol can cause irreparable damage to the viral proteins. As I explained earlier, proteins are defined by their 3D shape. When placed in different chemical environments (the higher pH's of soap) the shapes of these proteins can change irreparably (technically known as denaturation) and they will no longer work as intended.

Both soap and ethanol will kill the virus in a few seconds, yet government guidance advises washing your hands for 20 seconds, 30 seconds or even longer in different countries. This is more than enough time to kill the virus, so is the government advice wrong? No, but the point of washing your hands for that long is not that it takes that amount of time to kill the virus, but rather that people need to be encouraged to wash their hands for longer periods of time to ensure that they wash their entire hands. If the advice was to wash your hands for 2 seconds people would simply give their hands a quick wipe on the front and maybe the back, missing between the fingers, the thumbs and nails. Personally I would recommend watching Arnold Schwarzenegger's home video about hand washing which is both technically correct and features his pet donkey. You couldn't make this up. I can also tell you that in laboratory settings when testing for the coronavirus in patient samples we would regularly clean every surface with both soapy water and ethanol. It is common practice in such environments to coat with the disinfectant and wait a minimum of 3 minutes before treating the area as clean. In real world samples there is more to worry about than just coronavirus and it can take several minutes to kill off some of the more resistant viruses and bacteria that we can come into contact with, so it is best to follow the government advice and wash your hands for at least 30 seconds, and there is no harm in going for longer. Also be aware that continually washing your hands and using hand sanitizer can dry out the skin, moisturizing hand creams can help if your skin is getting dry and itchy.

### Self-isolating and lockdowns

Self-isolating is a new word for a very old concept. Restricting the movements of people to halt or restrict the spreading of disease always used to be called quarantining. For some reason though the terms "self-isolating" and "lockdown" are more commonly used when referring to the coronavirus pandemic. Perhaps they sound more friendly. The concept of quarantines is the oldest and least sophisticated way of dealing with the outbreak of any disease, if people don't see and interact with one another, then the virus cannot spread between them. If the virus is confined to a small group of people then hopefully they will all get the virus, recover and any virions die out before they re-join the wider population. The word quarantine originates from Venice and translates to 40 days. In the 1300s when ships would arrive in Venice they had to undergo a mandatory 40-day berth in the harbour, during which sailors were not allowed to disembark from their ships. Originally brought in to combat the black death which killed 30% of Europe's population between 1348 and 1359, but in those days it was actually a "trentine", lasting only 30 days. It was extended to 40 days in 1448 to combat the bubonic plague, which could take up to 37 days from infection to kill the host. By all accounts it was quite effective and the name has stuck.

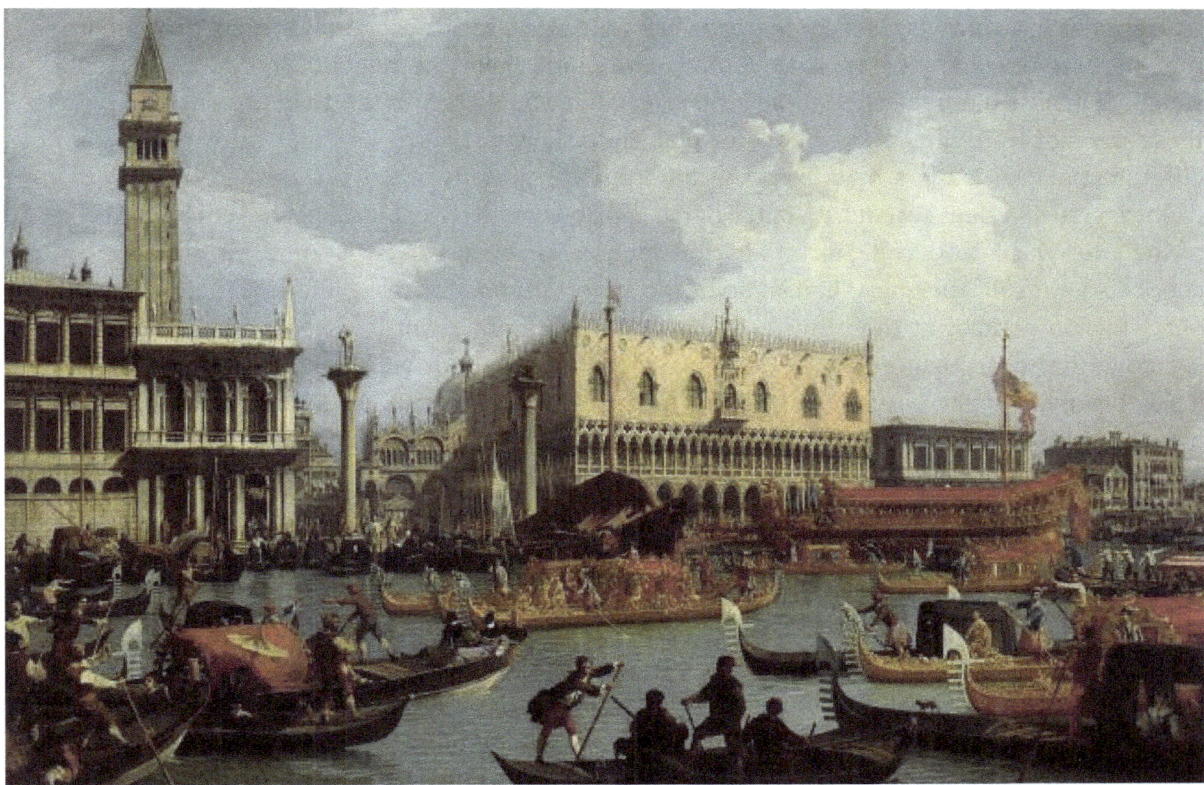

Although the venetians invented the term "quarantine" there are examples of sick individuals being isolated from human contact as far back as records go, with some references even appearing in the bible.[1] Perhaps the coolest fact about quarantines is that every astronaut who has ever been to the moon has been quarantined upon arrival back on Earth, including the Apollo 11 astronauts. Because no one had been to the moon there was a risk that the astronauts may bring back contagious life forms. So if you are sitting in your house now feeling down about the lockdowns, maybe it will help to know that you are in the same boat as astronauts.

So what anyone who is self-isolating really wants to know is this, does it work? The answer is yes, when done properly the evidence all shows that the spread of any virus is reduced by lockdowns. Proper lockdowns that people obey and that are sufficiently long do help prevent the spread of the virus. Lockdowns definitely reduce the human to human spread of the virus. There will always be some

---

[1] Isaiha 26:20 "Go, my people, enter your rooms and shut the doors behind you; hide yourselves for a little while until his wrath has passed by."

person to person spreading as it is almost impossible to keep everyone completely isolated. But the main way that the virus can infect people during lockdowns is by surviving on surfaces that multiple people touch and waiting for the lockdown to end. Without the lockdown the virus can spread by both methods. So it absolutely spreads less when a lockdown is in place, but some transfer always occurs. The evidence for this is to look at the "R numbers" within countries before during and after lockdowns. R numbers are the average number of people each infected person will go on to infect. For instance, if the R number is 2, then each person who is infected will go on to infect a further 2 people. Left unabated, cov-19 has an R number of about 3. However, during lockdowns in the UK the R number was reported to have dropped to about 0.6 to 0.9. Proving that the lockdowns do reduce the spread of the virus. An R number below 1 means that the number of people who have SARS-coV-2 is decreasing. R numbers are calculated by looking at the change in the number of positive cases over time.

Quarantines have always been controversial because of the social, economic and political implications that shutting down a geographic region raise. At some point the rights of individuals needs to be weighed against the public health benefits of a quarantine. More often than not in today's society, these decisions are left in the hands of politicians. It is not surprising that in different countries different political leaders have come to different conclusions about the best approach. In some countries, such a New Zealand, an initial harsh lockdown with strict measures to eliminate the spread of the virus was introduced. Since then, the country has been very strict on cross border migration checks. As a result, they have had some of the lowest number of cases in the world; only 474 cases per 1 million people. At the other end of the spectrum are countries like Sweden where no hard lockdown has ever been in place. There are many myths about why Sweden has never gone into lockdown, there are actually several reasons for this. Primarily though, the Swedish parliament doesn't actually have the authority to impose a lockdown. The Swedish constitution prevents the government declaring a state of emergency for anything other than war. As a result, Swedish case numbers have been much higher than other Scandinavian countries 64 820 cases per 1 million people (Denmark: 36 209, Finland: 10 170, Norway: 12 910 cases per 1 million people). For most countries however, what has actually been going in is an attempted compromise between the two extremes. This compromise takes the form of periods of locking down and gradual re-opening. With different countries (and sometimes cities or municipalities) having different tiers or ranking systems. Sometimes numbered, sometimes coloured. Coming in and out of different sets of restrictions as they try to balance the need for quarantine against public "covid fatigue" and the economic impact of lockdowns. The downside to trying to compromise on an issue like this is that the virus does not compromise. If you give it the chance to spread, it will. Most of the restrictions implemented in countries that compromise on the quarantine restrictions are not intended to eliminate the virus, but rather slow the spread to prevent the complete overwhelming and collapse of the health service.

One final matter that should be discussed on the topic of lockdown are the mental health issues that arise as a result of self-isolation. Several studies have found a substantial increase in reports of depression, insomnia, post-traumatic stress disorder, anxiety and stress during lockdowns. With anywhere between 15-40 % of those questioned reporting one or more of the above feelings. Most studies also show that women seem to be suffering more than men during lockdowns. There is no scientific explanation for why women would suffer more than men, although there is still a pervasive stigma attached to men discussing issues of mental health and that can often account for these trends in the data. There is a definite and undeniable correlation between being poor, and poorer mental health in all these statistics. Those with nicer houses to quarantine in and plenty of savings in the bank are not suffering as much as those who have less. Which just goes to show that the old saying was wrong; money can buy you happiness.

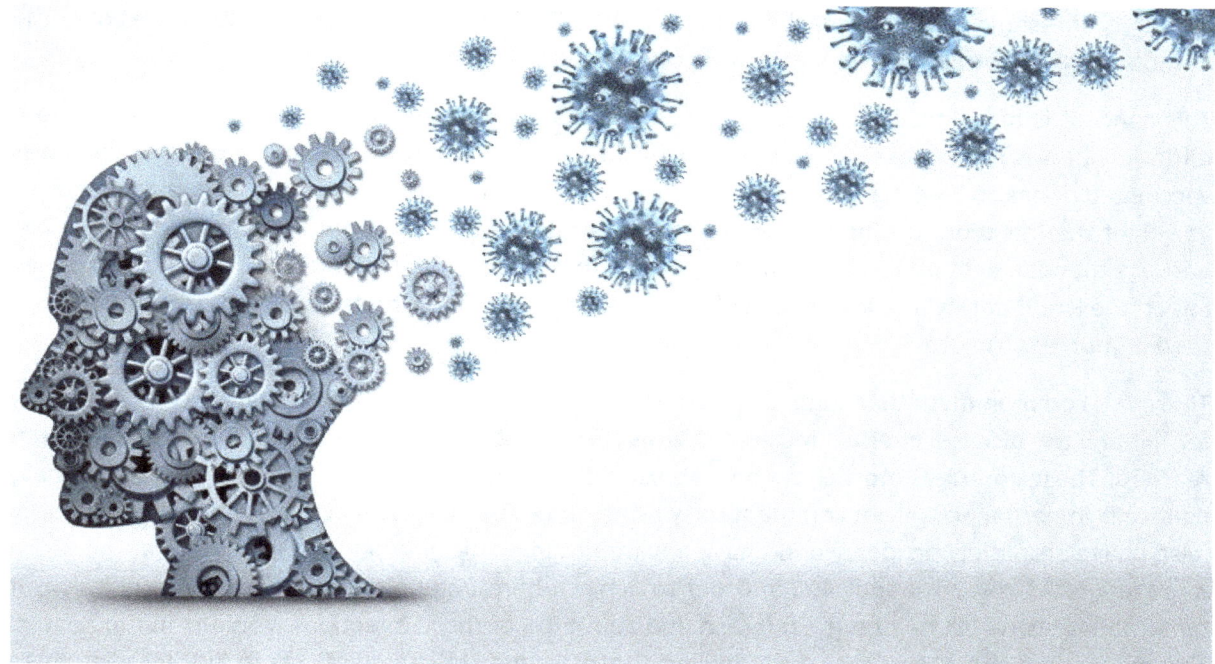

One of the biggest worries when it comes to the mental wellbeing of people during a lockdown is that it may lead to an increase in suicide. Thankfully, the data has shown that this has not happened. In a study on the suicide rates in Japan, there was actually a 14% decrease in the number of suicides recorded during the first months (Feb-Jun 2020) of lockdowns being introduced. However, as the second wave of the virus hit and more restrictions were put in place, there was a 16% increase, taking the number back up to just above where they were pre-pandemic. These data are not restricted to Japan but have been largely observed worldwide. The explanation for this may be that during the first lockdown, people were generally working less than they had been before, they had government subsidies and were spending more time at home with their families; generally enjoying a better work life balance than they had been before, resulting in a sharp decrease in suicides.[2] However when the second lockdown came in, and the full economic impact started to hit, with job losses, financial insecurity and boredom as life became more monotonous, the number of suicides began to increase again, but not significantly above what they were pre-pandemic…yet. It is an unfortunate statistic that being unemployed increases someone's risk of committing suicide two to threefold. As the job losses due to corona increase there is a real fear that the suicide rates will too.

## Herd immunity

Most people will have never heard of herd immunity before the pandemic. This is a concept by which epidemiologists (scientists who study the progression and spread of diseases in the human population) reckon that if a certain percentage of the population (thought to be about 60-75% for covid-19) are immune to a virus, they will prevent or slow the spread of the virus to those who aren't immune. Conceptually this means that if enough people have immunity, the virus cannot go through them to infect someone new. Perhaps this is best explained with an example. Imagine a classroom with 20 students, all of whom have been vaccinated. Their teacher has never had SARS-cov-2 or been vaccinated. If one of the children´s family members was to get sick, the virus would need to jump from the family member, to the child and then to the teacher. If the child is vaccinated, then this path from the family member to the teacher is more difficult than if the child is not vaccinated. Once the herd

---

[2] Which should make us question our pre-pandemic lifestyles.

immunity threshold has been reached (this is the 60-75% of the population mentioned above) the number of cases within the population will gradually decrease to 0.

This concept is often misunderstood. It can slow the spread of the virus and make that path more difficult, but it is not impossible for that teacher to get the virus *via* the child. Even if that child was vaccinated or has an T-cells and B-cells, if they get the virus it will take some time for these to mobilise and fight the infection. During this period the child may be able to spread the virus to others, but because they can fight off an infection faster than if they had no immunity, the number of people they infect (the R number) will be lower. As with other forms of immunity, mutations of the virus can render herd immunity obsolete.

There is a common myth that some governments are attempting to use herd immunity as a strategy for fighting the disease. In effect letting the virus spread until the herd immunity threshold had been reached. Those countries most commonly accused of this are the U.K. and Sweden. I want to remain politically impartial, so will not comment on whether or not this was ever actually a government policy (also I have absolutely no idea, I don't have any friends in politics). What I would say is that the death rate from SARS-cov-2 is about 4%. In order to achieve herd immunity 60-75% of the population of these countries would need to be infected and about 4% of those infections would result in deaths. This means that there would be 1.6-2 million deaths in the U.K. and 250 000 to 300 000 deaths in Sweden. The total number of deaths in each country are currently much lower than this (123 000 in the U.K. and 12 000 in Sweden). So if they were going for herd immunity, it hasn't worked.

# Testing for covid-19

## PCR tests

PCR tests are the golden standard for any type of nucleic acid (DNA or RNA) test. The specific type of PCR test being used for covid-19 is an "RT-qPCR" test. PCR tests allow us to directly detect the coronavirus itself, both within and outside of human cells. The test can even be used for detecting the virus on surfaces. It does so by looking for sequences of RNA that are specific to (only ever found in) this specific coronavirus. If you have a positive RT-qPCR test result, you absolutely have the virus and are contagious as the virus is present wherever you tested. I will discuss swabbing and other testing methods below. This test cannot tell you if you have had the virus and have recovered.

So what is an RT-qPCR test? Well, for starters, RT-qPCR is an acronym for "Reverse Transcription Quantitative Polymerase Chain Reaction". Transcription is a biological process in which a DNA sequence is copied to make its corresponding RNA sequence. For example, if a DNA sequence reads as follows:

ATCG

It would be transcribed and a short strand of RNA with the following sequence will be made:

UAGC

These two sequences are said to be "complimentary" as they will bind to each other. An "A" will always bind to a "T" (or "U" if it is RNA instead of DNA) and a "G" will always bind to a "C" to make a double helix. In this case we are testing for a retrovirus, so we are putting RNA into the test which means it needs to be converted to DNA. The first step of an RT-qPCR test is a "reverse transcription" in which the RNA in the sample is converted to DNA. This is done using enzymes found in nature called, imaginatively, "reverse transcriptases". There is a tendency in biology to name enzymes after what they do, which is quite handy. The DNA made from, and complementary to, RNA is called cDNA (literally complementary DNA). The second part of this test, the bit that comes after the hyphen, is where the real magic happens.

"DNA amplification" is a process in which a strand of DNA with a specific sequence is copied to make two copies with the exact same sequence. In order to do this the samples must first be heated to about 95 °C. At this temperature the chemical bonds holding the two strands that make up DNA are broken and the strands split. This is usually referred to as "single stranded DNA" (ssDNA). When the sample is cooled, the two DNA strands will want to bind back together. However, if we put in a short, man-made ssDNA that is complimentary (has the sequence that will bind to a part of one of the strands) it will bind to the DNA rather than the original strand. We also have an enzyme called Taq polymerase (whose discovery won a Nobel prize in 1993) and all the building blocks to make more DNA added to the solution being tested. When the temperature is cooled down to 72 °C this amazing little enzyme starts to make more DNA at the end of the short man made sequence (known as a primer) using the original longer strand as a template. By this I mean that wherever there is an "A" on the original sequence it will put a T on the new strand and *vice versa*. The chemical name for any reaction in which a few small chemicals are built into a long chain is a "polymerisation reaction".[3] Hence the enzyme is called a polymerase and we get the "P" in PCR. The Taq in the enzyme name refers to *"Thermus aquaticus",* the bacteria in which the enzyme was discovered.

---

[3] The same type of reaction is used to make plastics, which is why they are called polymers.

## Polymerase chain reaction - PCR

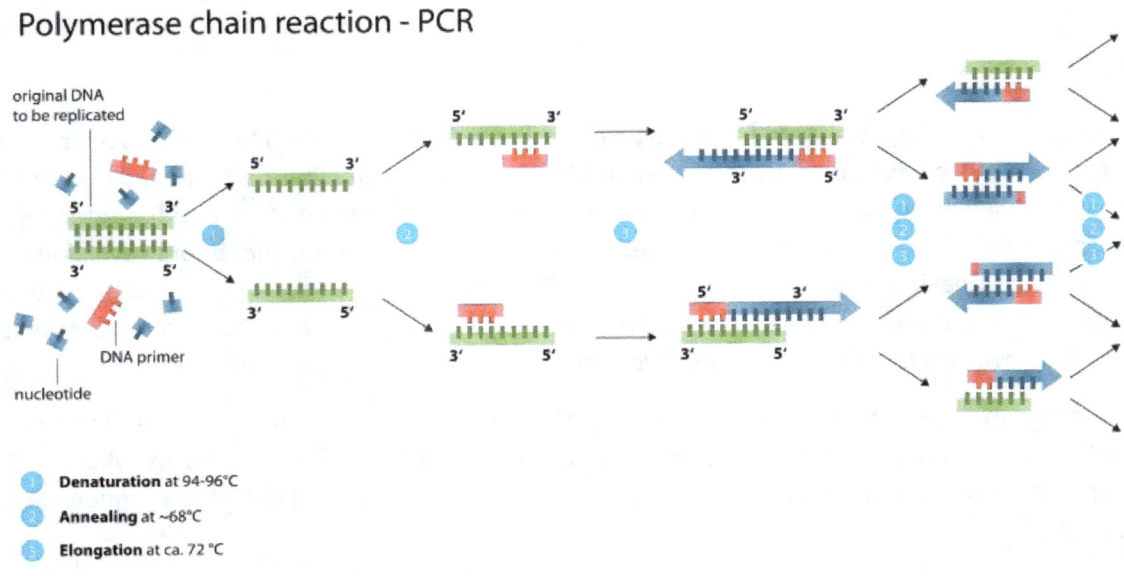

If we start with a single strand of RNA, the reverse transcription will create a cDNA strand which is bound to the original RNA sequence. We now have a double stranded sequence of all the RNA in the sample. Next, we heat the sample to 95 °C, then cool to 72 °C; to force the double strands to break apart and then come back together. Although usually they will bind to a short sequence of DNA we have put into the reaction that will specifically bind to DNA sequences specific to the virus. Polymerases will then create more DNA around the synthetic DNA we added. Since both strands are amplified this way, what started off as one double stranded DNA has now become two double strands of DNA with the exact same sequence. By repeating this process, the amount of DNA can be very quickly and easily increased. Each repetition of heating and cooling is referred to as a "cycle", and each cycle will double the amount of DNA present.

That is the basic process by which RT-PCR works. It is extremely accurate, Taq polymerase will make on average, 1 mistake in every 100 000 000 to 1 000 000 000 DNA bases that it copies. I told you it was magic. Now comes the really cool part, where we put the "q" into qPCR. So far all I have really explained is how we can make more DNA from some initial starting RNA. The question remains though how we actually detect how much DNA we have.

This is done using a technique called "fluorescence", literally emitting light. Remember the primers I mentioned earlier (the short man made sequences of DNA). They are the most important part of all PCR tests, but especially important for qPCR. These are designed to be about 13-30 bases long, this is long enough to have a sequence specific to what is being tested for, in this case the covid-19 virus. Yes, the sequence that we test for is only about 20 bases long and that specific sequence of 20 bases is not found anywhere else in nature than in the coronavirus. Primers in qPCR are even more special in that they are designed and made with a "fluorophore" at one end of the strand and a "quencher" at the other. Fluorophores are chemicals that emit light, literally shine one colour, like glow sticks. A quencher is a molecule that stops the fluorophore from emitting light. Quenchers only work when they are held in close proximity to the fluorophore. The primers are short enough that having a fluorophore at one end and quencher at the other keeps them close enough that no light is given out. When the primer binds to the DNA being amplified the polymerase enzyme starts to elongate the primers, the fluorophore is kicked off and floats away into solution. In doing so it now gets further away from the quencher and can start to emit light. We can then easily measure the amount of light emitted by a sample and calculate not only if there was RNA with a sequence only found in covid-19, but how much there was. Remember, each "cycle" doubles the amount of DNA in the sample and we know the smallest amount of light we can measure, so this calculation is actually fairly easy. The "limit of detection", the smallest amount of RNA that can be detected by RT-qPCR depends on the quality of primers, but can be as low as being able to detect a single virion in the sample tested.

In practice each sample is assigned a "Ct" value. If you keep cycling eventually the amplification will stop because you have used up all the primers in the solution or the amount of light being produced is more than the machine (called a thermocycler) can measure. The Ct value is the number of cycles it takes to reach half of this maximum. I have included my own data below from tests done when I was negative and positive for coronavirus. In them you can see that my Ct values are Ct=X. You will notice that there are two curves on the positive result and one on the negative result. A control built into the testing is to also detect a sequence of DNA found in all human beings. If this showed no result it would mean that the swab had no human DNA on it, which usually means the swabbing was not done properly. The lowest value we ever saw for any samples when testing for corona was a Ct of 13. Which means we only had to double the amount of RNA in the sample 13 times to get a high signal, Ct values above "34ish" are treated as inconclusive or negative and there is never any need to do more than 40 cycles. The average time to run a PCR is about 90 minutes, but there are lots of steps before and after that make it take longer. Modern PCR machines, known as thermocyclers, can run either 96 or 384 samples at once, some of which will be controls.

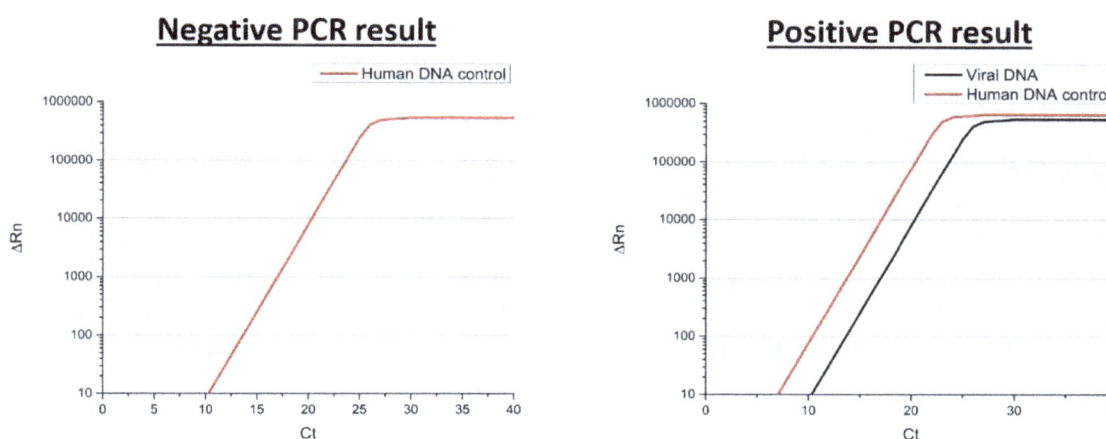

Please do not ask your local test centre for your own personal Ct values. They are overworked and stressed as it is and do not have the time to respond to such requests. Also the number is a little meaningless on its own as you will have different amounts of viral DNA on two swabs taken at the same time just through random chance. Also your samples are treated with the highest level of confidentiality so your data cannot be disclosed and those testing you are not allowed to know who each sample belongs to.

I realise that this section may be a bit confusing, I have gone to some effort to make the concept more understandable using images. Bear in mind that PCR is a complicated technique that people spend years understanding and perfecting. There is no shame in not understanding exactly how it works, however, what is important is to know that PCR tests can detect viral RNA with extreme sensitivity and are very reliable. PCR is an incredibly robust technique used daily in research, diagnostic, commercial and forensic labs around the world. For instance, genealogy companies such as 23 and me® do PCR using primers specific to DNA sequences that only appear from different geographical locations at different points of time in human evolution. The underlying science is rock solid and issues with the tests are always either a result of human error or issues in the diagnostic pipeline.

## The diagnostic pipeline

There are many firsts as a result of the coronavirus pandemic. PCR was only developed in the 1980s, so this is the first truly global pandemic that we as a species have faced and been able to test for using PCR. Whilst the technology has been widely available and utilised for decades, being able to test on this scale has never been attempted before and has required some incredibly hard work from lots of talented and hardworking individuals. I will now go through each step of the diagnostic pipeline, explaining how each part works and common issues that arise and how to avoid them.

## The test kits

So the kits that arrive at your door or that the nurse testing you will use have to be put together. This is done by teams of people working around the clock trying to source all the component parts from different suppliers. They also need to monitor the age and quality of some of the kit components, as they can expire. Every test kit should contain instructions on how to use it, a vial or tube with a liquid in it and a paper towel; all sealed in a clear plastic bag. In most cases, but not all, the test will also contain a swab. This last sentence may surprise many people, but swabbing is not the only method of getting a sample. Every kit has to be packed and sent out by people in very clean conditions wearing personal protective equipment (PPE). Otherwise a single person packing kits who has corona may unwittingly contaminate the kits they are packing and send thousands of contaminated kits to those being tested, spreading the infection.

Let´s begin with the instructions, these are not the same in different parts of the world. Even within a single country the instructions can differ between cities and regions. One by-product of this is that it is extremely difficult to compare data from different regions as the quality of the sampling is different. For example, in Sweden the average Ct values are lower (which means more RNA is found on each swab) in Stockholm than they are in Gothenburg. The reason for this is that the instructions sent out with the Stockholm kits tell people to swab their throats, noses and spit onto the swab. The instructions in Gothenburg just ask people to swab their throats, so they will, on average, have less viral RNA on the swabs. You should follow the instructions provided with your kit, please do not do anything differently based on what is written here. Your tests have been validated and will work as instructed.

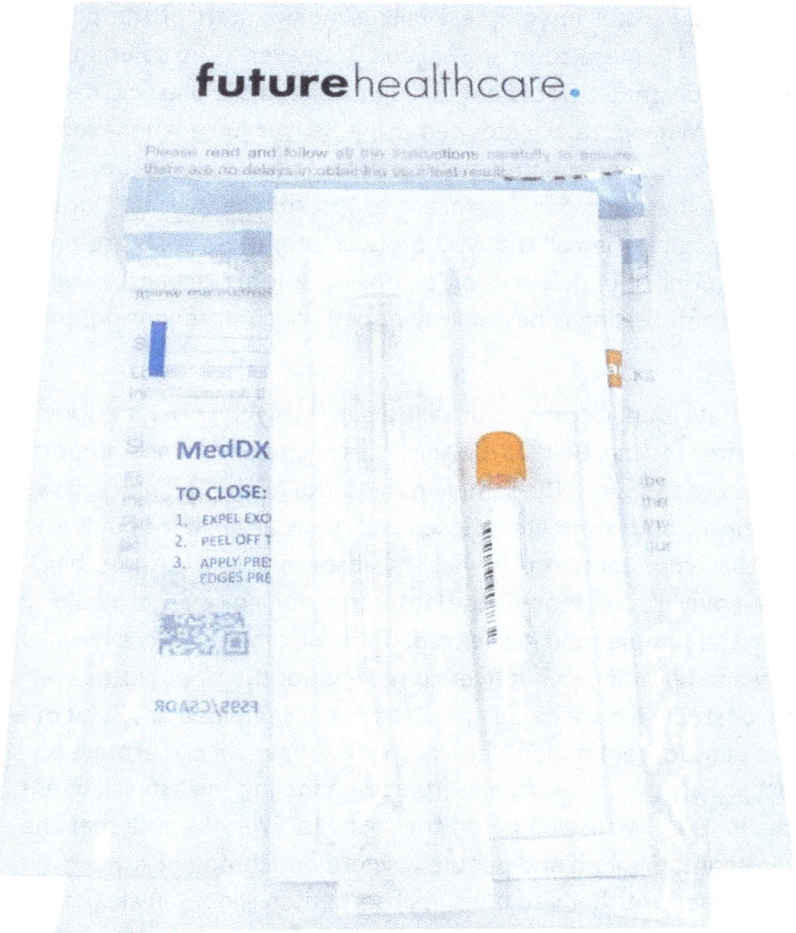

The next thing you will find in the test kit is the vial or tube containing a liquid. Tubes of any sort are in extremely short supply globally and testing centres are using anything they can get their hands on, so don't be surprised if you test several times and the tubes are different each time. On the outside of the tube there will be a label or a barcode or sticker of some kind. This is used to link your result to you. Please be sure to follow the instructions and link your test as required, otherwise you will not get a result. Every day we would get tens to hundreds of notes included with home test kits from people who weren't able to link their tests, sending us their personal phone numbers, addresses or emails to try and get their results. Unfortunately for these people, their samples were discarded; literally put in bins to be incinerated. Testing centres are running beyond full capacity with people regularly working 16-20 hours a day and there simply is not the time to track and report the results of the couple of hundred unregistered samples received daily. In the time it would take to call and report a single result that staff member could test another 100 samples that have been registered. That being said, I would like to take the opportunity to personally thank those people who included thank you notes in their test kits, it does brighten up the days of those working in the testing centres. An extra special thanks should also be extended to the one person who put a tip of 20 sek in their test kit. This was extremely well received.

Inside the vials is a small amount of liquid. What is in this liquid will vary between countries but it is not just water. It contains a special solution designed to stabilise the DNA in your sample and keep it viable whilst being transported to the testing centre. Please do not drink it, throw it out or top it up with tap water. This could result in your test failing. At the start of the pandemic in Sweden the solution was supplied by a Chinese company called "Dr Beaver". The solution, lovingly referred to as "beaver juice" was so acidic that it would eat through some of the plastic covers we put on top of the samples at a later step. We eventually stopped using beaver juice whenever possible, it in no way made the PCR not work but meant that none of the samples could be stored for later studies. Please bear in mind that these samples are meant to test for the virus in your nose and or throat. As lovely as the other "biological media" that you produce are; these tests are not designed to test for the coronavirus in your urine, blood, faeces or (on one occasion) ejaculate. How and why people insist on sending these things for testing is beyond my powers of comprehension; but if you are tempted, please don't.

All test kits should contain is an absorbent, usually a paper towel. This is not for you to blow your nose or wipe your mouth after testing. Believe it or not, this is one of the most important parts of the test kit. The absorbent is there to show if the sample has leaked. All the samples are sent out in clear plastic bags that should be firmly and completely closed with your used kit inside. It is important (actually a legal requirement) that your sample tube has an absorbent in the same bag. When we come to opening and testing your kits we look at the absorbent for any sign of liquid on it. The absorbent should only be wet if the sample tube has leaked. If the absorbent looks even slightly wet the sample will be thrown away and burned without ever coming out of the clear plastic bag. This is not us being unnecessarily harsh or strict. We are handling thousands of samples a day, a lot of which have a deadly virus inside. That bit of absorbent paper is one of the few ways we can protect ourselves from directly coming into contact with the virus. Also, if the person handling the sample opens a leaked tube that has the coronavirus in it, the virus will be on their gloves. Every sample that they handle after that runs the risk of being contaminated and people who are not corona positive may get positive results. It is therefore vitally important that you put the absorbent in the same clear plastic bag as your tube and close the bag and tube properly. Another common mistake is people wrapping the tubes in the absorbent, if the tube is only leaking a little there might not be enough liquid to go all the way through the absorbent, so the sample needs to be unwrapped from the absorbent in the clear bag, which is quite difficult and time consuming. As a general rule of thumb, the kit should look the same when you send it back as it did when you received it, except for without the swab.

## Swabbing (Nasopharyngeal swabs)

Now to the infamous swabs. It may surprise some to know that not all tests include swabs. This is not because the users are expected to provide their own; but rather they are not needed. In Vienna for example, swab less tests are used, in which the patients gargle a solution which they then spit back into the tubes which are sent off for analysis. I'm sure that those reading this who have gone through the discomfort of a nasopharyngeal swab test might be upset by this fact. There are countless accounts of people being hurt and in pain for days, with swabs stuck through their nostrils to the back of their throats: there are even viral videos of people testing themselves, and we know for a fact that people are making themselves vomit when testing, because there is vomit in some of the sample tubes we receive. This is all completely unnecessary. Don't get me wrong, the testing should be uncomfortable, but in no way should you be in pain when testing. Such as one Swedish man who had to have a swab that broke surgically removed from his nasal cavity. Now I have had arguments with other trained professionals about this and these are my own views and you should always follow the advice on the instructions provided with your kit. But in my opinion, this virus can get from one person to another in high enough quantities to infect and kill millions of people around the world just from breathing it out and travelling through the air. That means there must be quite a lot of the virus in your throat, mouth and nose. The RT-qPCR tests are extremely sensitive. If you put a swab to the back of your throat and wiggle for a couple of seconds, you are bound to get enough on it to detect any virus that is there. Also the tests have in built fail-safes with the human DNA test. If your sample has no DNA in it, you will be sent another test to take. In practice, all that is needed is to roll the swabs at the back of the throat where it feels uncomfortable for a couple of seconds. Some regions also require the swabbing of the nose. You do not need to poke the swab up to your brain. If you are contagious the virus will be present in your nose in high numbers. It should be uncomfortable because you want to make absolutely sure you have got as much virus on the swab as possible to get a good result but please do not cause yourself any pain in testing.

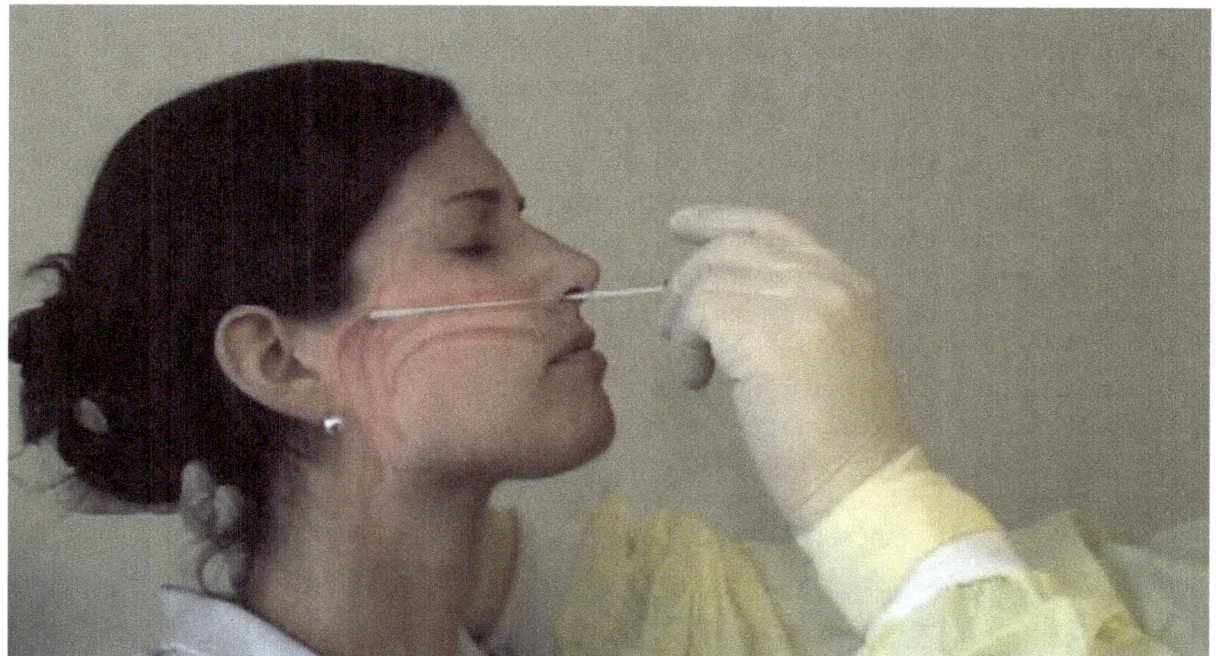

Please do not test each other, this is illegal, for several reasons. First you could seriously hurt the person being test, secondly if you are being tested it should be because you think you might have the virus and should be self-isolating so shouldn't be coming into contact with anyone until you get your test results. We had several instances where people doing at home tests would test their children then phoned the test centre telling us these were children's test results. Presumably so we would expedite or take more care with the tests or send the results directly to the parents. Whenever this happened the samples were binned and the parents warned not to test their children again. If children need tested the test should be performed by someone trained to administer the test safely.

Once you have used the swab, if the instructions tell you to leave the swab in the tube then please do so, however, they usually do not. Normally the procedure is to swirl the end of the swab in the test solution then take the swab out and throw it in the bin. If you leave the swab in when you shouldn't that means that someone has to take it out, which takes time. Whilst this might not sound like a big deal, when you are testing thousands of samples a day it does add up. Also a lot of sample processing is done using robots, if there is a swab in a sample tube and someone misses it, the robot can crash into the swab and break. The robot will then need to be fixed and the samples in the robot normally need to be re-run. All of which slows down a pipeline running at full tilt to keep up with demand.

In order to get around this most testing centres that do not want swabs left in the tubes will try to send out kits with swabs that are too big to fit in the vials. To make people think twice and check the instructions before sending the sample back. Despite this, some people will still bend or break the swabs, determined to get them into the tubes. Please don´t be one of those people. Another common mistake is to put the swab back into the clear bag with the sample tube. Unfortunately, since that swab has been used, it has now contaminated the entire inside of the bag. Your test tube included, so the entire thing will be discarded for the safety of those handling it and to prevent contamination of other samples.

So those are the test kits and how to use them. But once a test has been taken what happens to it?

## Logistics

Getting the test kits out to people, and then back to the testing centre sounds pretty straightforward. In fact, it has some pretty serious challenges. Samples of this nature should be packed in clear boxes with an absorbent material inside. This is done so that upon receiving them, the staff at the testing centre can see if any of the samples have leaked into the box before opening it and potentially exposing themselves to the samples. These boxes are then transported to the testing centre by plane, train, automobile or foot depending on where the nearest testing centre is. Transporting this number of samples over such large distances is expensive and time consuming. As a result, some countries have favoured drive in test centres, where those who need tested never leave their cars and are tested through their windows. These centres can in theory cover more people who can drive larger distances to the test centres. However not everyone has a car or live large distances from any test centres. In these instances, the test kits need to be dropped off at people's houses, they test themselves and the drivers take the tests back to the test centre. All of which is expensive and time consuming. Especially when 10% of those who book tests don´t have the common decency to even be at home when their test kits arrive. If you don't need a test don't book one, if you need a test you should be self-isolating in your home anyway and there is no excuse for missing a pre-booked test.

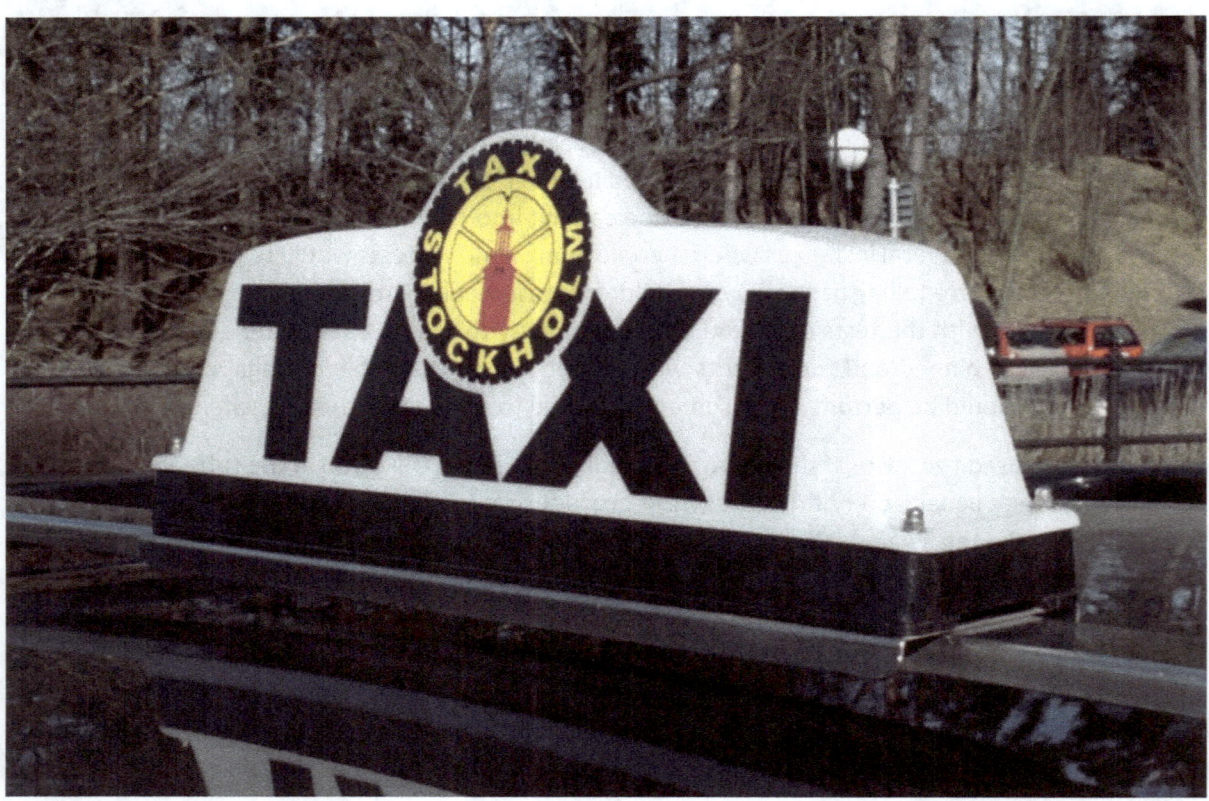

One interesting solution that was done in Stockholm during the pandemic was to get taxi drivers involved. With more people working from home and self-isolating, taxi drivers have seen a drastic decrease in their business. By hiring them to deliver test kits to people´s homes and bring them to the centre on the same day, taxi drivers were kept in work and a lot of the logistics issues were resolved. All in all, quite a clever solution to the problem.

## At the testing centre

Once the samples arrive at the testing centre they are normally put into a cold storage room until they can be dealt with if there is a backlog. Each sample is then opened by hand and "inactivated" to make it safe to handle. Inactivation is a process in which any virus or pathogen in the sample is "killed" in a way that does not compromise the intended test. For covid-19 testing there are several ways of doing this, either by adding chemicals such as detergents, by irradiating with UV lamps or by heating in ovens. Once inactivated the samples are normally pipetted into special plates that allow multiple samples to be processed simultaneously before the RNA is "extracted" from the samples. The samples will contain intact human cells and virions which must be broken open so that the RNA and DNA inside of them falls out (a process called lysis). However, biological samples contain lots of things other than DNA/RNA. We therefore also need to clean up the samples to remove all the unwanted proteins and other nasty stuff. There are lots of different ways to get the RNA and DNA out of the samples: some pipelines use chemical methods such as salts, ethanol and detergents; other labs use magnetic beads and grind and break open the cells and virions. This is done by violently shaking the samples with the beads inside and using beads that will preferentially stick to RNA and DNA over all the other stuff in the sample. This method allows the samples to be washed as well by holding the beads in place with a strong magnet and flowing a wash solution over them.

Once the RNA and DNA has been extracted from the sample it can be added to all the enzymes and other chemicals needed for RT-qPCR and reaction is started. Once the data has been gathered it then needs to be checked by trained staff and the results reported to the patients or doctors (if the patient is in hospital). In most countries, positive cases are also reported to relevant health authorities and track and trace programmes or mobile apps. This way, anyone who may have come into contact with someone who tests positive for the virus can be notified and put on alert to look for symptoms or get tested themselves. The computing and programming power involved in the diagnostic pipeline is simultaneously one of its biggest advantages and flaws. At every stage of the process the samples are tracked digitally and results can be reported very quickly using mobile technology. In some ways we are very lucky that this pandemic has struck at this point in history, even ten or fifteen years ago the technology available was not good enough to support the pipeline as it exists today. However, having everything digital means that we are in ways over reliant on the technology and when it encounters problems the entire pipeline is compromised. There were several days when the servers had problems or even the local internet went down and we were unable to process samples. Also these systems fail to protect the people most at risk of the virus. Elderly people do not understand the technology and are less likely to own smartphones so usually need to visit a testing or health centre in person to have their samples digitally registered by a nurse or doctor who gets their results and then contacts them. This increases the chance of infection as they come into contact with more people and it takes them longer to get results.

Another key task at the testing centres is to "sequence" some of the positive samples. Sequencing is a process by which the entire genetic sequence of the samples is determined. There are several ways of doing this and entire books have been written just on different sequencing methods. The purpose of sequencing is to look for mutations in the virus and to see how different clades (variants) are spreading geographically.

## Possible issues with PCR tests

So if the swabbing is done properly and there are no human errors in the pipeline, RT-qPCR tests work perfectly. Scientifically these are extremely robust tests, if something goes wrong it is always because a person made a mistake. There are in fact three possible results from a PCR test. "Negative" - no viral RNA present in the sample, "Positive" - viral RNA present and "inconclusive". Inconclusive refers to samples that need to be retaken because something has gone wrong in the pipeline.

The first and most obvious mistake is that the swab has not been taken properly. However, since there is an inbuilt control to test for human DNA sequences. You would literally need to have not touched your throat with the swab at all to have any chance of this failing. So there are inbuilt controls and the samples will be failed if the swabbing is not done properly. Anecdotally, this is very rare.

The primers used in RT-PCR are designed to be specific to the virus. A lot of work goes into finding sequences that are only found in the viral genome and that are suitable for use as PCR primers. However, the virus is constantly evolving and if there is a mutation in the sequence of viral RNA to which the primer binds then the virus may go undetected. The only known solution to this is to have several primers for the virus in each test solution. This increases the cost of each test at a time when the raw materials are in unprecedented demand and the global economy has taken a large hit. It is therefore rarely the case that two primers are the used. If there have been mutations in this region there is a good chance that people are who have infections are being incorrectly told they don't have covid-19. What is also worrying is that sequencing is only ever done on samples that test positive for covid-19 in a PCR test. If a variant with a mutation in the genetic sequence where the primer binds were to arise, and this mutation meant that the primer didn't bind and the PCR test didn't work, then we would have no way of detecting the variant. It is a real possibility that a variant could exist that we do not detect by PCR. The result of this would be that people who are positive are given a negative PCR result, and a variant of the virus would spread unknown. This would actually require several mutations within the 20 bases that the primers bind to, which makes it unlikely, but not impossible. If one base mutates the primers will typically still bind, just not as well. As more variants of the virus evolve, the chances of this happening are much greater.

## Antibody tests

Testing for Antibodies will, in theory, tell you if you have had an infection. It does not necessarily tell you if you have an active infection. This has caused some confusion amongst the general public, because the biology has not been properly communicated to them. In the chapter of this book on the immune response I explain that antibodies are made by B-cells, their main function is to bind to virions floating around outside of cells in your body; sticking to their spike proteins and preventing the virions from infecting more potential host cells. If you ever get re-infected, the antibodies specific to those spike proteins will get mass produced quickly and help fight off an infection faster than a new, unrecognised, pathogen. However, when you get sick for the first time it takes your B-cells hours to days (it varies from person to person) to be activated to start the process of manufacturing new antibodies for this infection. Even after activation it can take days or even weeks to select and then mass produce enough antibodies to fight and clear out the virus from your body. After clearing the virus, antibodies specific to cov-19 will still circulate around your body for several weeks to make sure all the virus has been completely cleared out and fight off a potential re-infection. On average the highest concentration of antibodies will be circulating in the patient's blood about three weeks after the initial infection. If you are planning on getting an antibody test this is the optimum time to do so since after this time the antibodies in your blood stream will gradually decrease. This is not the reason that you lose immunity over time. There are still those memory B-cells in the lymphatic system that can mass produce more B-cells and antibodies if another infection arises.

Most antibody tests will only be able to detect those antibodies in your blood stream for a few weeks after infection. After about 45-60 days they should fail, as these antibodies are cleared out of your bloodstream. They do not test for memory B-cells or T-cells. Having a negative antibody result does not necessarily mean that you did not have a cov-19 infection. Coupled with this the testing for antibodies is nowhere near as robust as the PCR tests and is fraught with difficulties and errors. This has led to most governments basically ignoring the results of antibody tests, they are not accepted as valid tests for travelling between countries. But how exactly do these tests work and what are the problems with them?

These are blood based tests, so a blood sample is required. It is, quite understandably, not possible for people to take and send in their own blood for testing. It is therefore necessary for those being tested to go to a local doctor's office or testing centre for a nurse or doctor to take a blood sample. Once they reach the test centre, the samples are "centrifuged", spun extremely quickly, to create centrifugal forces that separate out the different components of the blood. The speeds at which blood samples are spun literally pull the components of the sample at thousands of times the force of gravity. Under these conditions the heavier components (red blood cells) form a little pellet at the bottom of the sample tube, and the lighter, mostly water based, components float around within the tube. The antibodies are in the lighter top bit. The top solution is then carefully removed and taken on for further testing in a "lateral flow assay".

Lateral flow assays come in several forms but the basic way that they work is roughly the same. The basics of any lateral flow assay is that a testing surface is coated with either the virus itself or the spike proteins from the virus that have been artificially grown and purified in a lab. The centrifuged test solution from the sample is then flown over this surface from one side to another, hence the "lateral" (fancy way of saying from one side of the test to the other) and "flow" in "lateral flow assay". "Assay" is just a technical term for a test for a specific molecule from the immune system or the activity of a biological molecule. If you have any antibodies in your sample they will stick to the spike proteins on the test surface. Since antibodies are "Y" shaped with the top of the "Y" sticking to the spike protein, the bottom of the Y will be sticking out away from the surface. Luckily this is the "conserved" region of the antibody structure, which is the same on all antibodies of that type. Other antibodies have therefore been found that will bind to this conserved region of each antibody type. We call these secondary antibodies because they are the second antibodies in our test and are used to make "sandwich assays". Once the sample proteins have been run over the surface, if the sample has antibodies for the spike proteins they will stick to the surface. The sample is then rinsed to wash off all the other gunk in the sample that doesn't stick to the spike proteins, or any antibodies just lying loose on the surface. Secondary antibodies that will stick to the tails of antibodies are then flown over the surface before a final rinse step. These secondary antibodies are made in labs and designed to have chemical labels on them that have a colour of some sort. Therefore, when they stick to the antibodies stuck to the surface they will cause it to change colour. There is a diagram included that might be easier to follow than the text. Sometimes rather than a colour change a fluorescent chemical is attached to the secondary antibodies. Similar test have also now been developed to test for the presence of virions in a sample. These are known as lateral flow "antigen" tests, since the virus is considered the antigen.

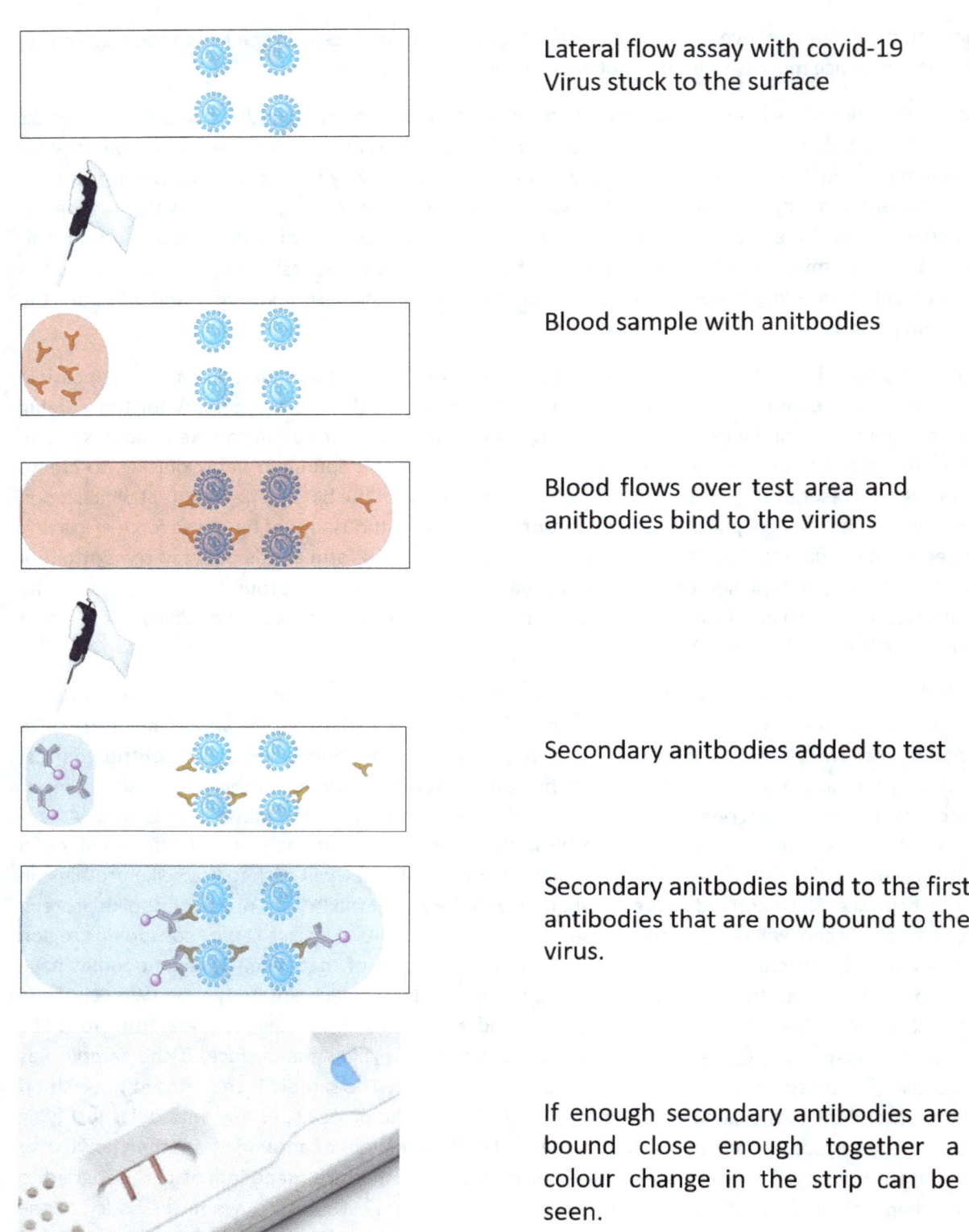

Lateral flow assay with covid-19 Virus stuck to the surface

Blood sample with anitbodies

Blood flows over test area and anitbodies bind to the virions

Secondary anitbodies added to test

Secondary anitbodies bind to the first antibodies that are now bound to the virus.

If enough secondary antibodies are bound close enough together a colour change in the strip can be seen.

Antibody tests are, for the most part, not needed. If you get sick and have a positive PCR test for cov-19 you have SARS-cov-2. If you get better, then you have almost definitely got T-cells, B-cells (and by virtue antibodies) that fought off the infection. The exception to this would be if your initial immune response was enough to fight off the infection. In either case why would you need an antibody test?

The only reason you would need an antibody test is if you were sick and unable to get a PCR test to confirm if you had SARS-cov-2.

The most common reason to take an antibody test is 3-4 weeks after vaccination to determine if you have produced antibodies that will bind to the covid-19 virus. In other words, to determine if the vaccine has given you immunity. When antibodies are first produced they are mass produced and circulate in your bloodstream for several weeks to months to fight off any more virus that gets into your system. However, over time their numbers fall off. Six months after a coronavirus infection most people will produce negative antibody test results. This does not mean they have no immunity, they could still have B-cell and T-cell immunity for the variant of the virus that they were infected with. How quickly your antibody count drops off after an infection differs from person to person, but you will usually have antibodies in your blood stream for 2-3 months at least after an infection. If you were sick 6 months ago and never got tested there is no way to determine if you had SARS-cov-2 or not.

Whilst these lateral flow tests are good, they are not always considered as proof of an infection, for the antibody tests this makes sense given that antibody biology is quite time dependant and complicated. For the antigen lateral flow assays, they are sometimes not considered good enough because they are not as reliable as the PCR tests.

## SARS-cov-2 treatments

At the moment there are no recognised treatments for SARS-cov-2. All that can be done to alleviate suffering in the most serious cases that require hospitalisation is to provide oxygen to make it easier for people to breathe and the practice of rotating those with severe pneumonia to spread the damage of the lungs and hopefully give the immune system enough time to clear the infection. That being said, several treatments have been tried.

### Remdesivir

Remdesivir is an antiviral drug developed by Gilead Sciences Ltd. It is administered by injection and is what is technically known as a "prodrug". Prodrugs are chemicals that are completely inactive as they are, but enzymes within your body will convert them into an active drug. The way remdesivir works, its "mode of action" is the technical term, is that it gets into your cells and is converted into a molecule similar to the RNA base adenosine (A). The polymerases in your cells that are making copies of the viral RNA will take up the active form of remdesivir and use it instead of adenosine. Only when they do so the drug will cause the replication to stop there. The RNA chain will not get any longer. As a result, viral RNA can no longer be properly made and virus production within the host cell is effectively stopped. Remdesivir was not developed specifically for cov-19 and has previously been sold to treat various viruses including ebola and hepatitis C.

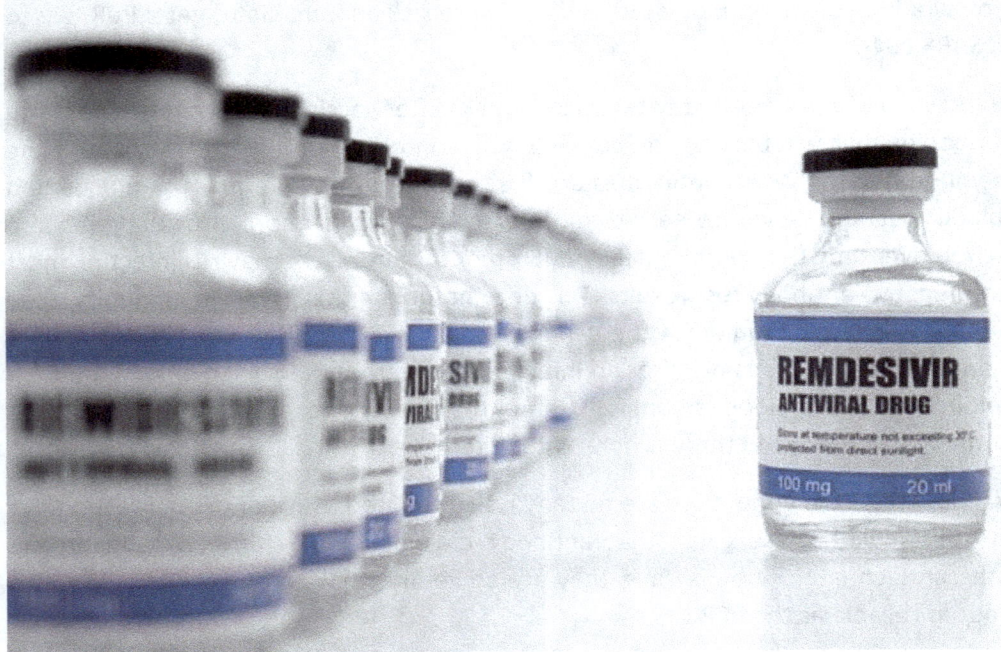

Remdesivir is a very controversial drug. It is currently only approved for use in the most serious cases of SARS-cov-2 and even then only in 50 countries. There are several reasons for this. The first is that it is debatable whether or not it works. The initial studies showed that Remdesivir could shorten the average time a patient with SARS-cov-2 spent in intensive care from 15 days to 10 days and improve the life expectancy of those who got the treatment, with 11.9% of those in intensive care who didn't get the drug dying within 15 days, whereas only 6.7% of those who did get the drug dying in the same time period. However, later studies showed that the drug had no impact whatsoever on patient outcomes. So what happened? Did the virus evolve to combat the drug? I'm afraid the answer is much more depressing. The initial studies were at best biased or at worst flat out fraud. In any study like this, the scientists who conduct and publish the work are required to disclose who actually funded the study. In these initial trials of remdesivir, the work was not funded by Gilead but by the centre for disease control (CDC); if pharmaceutical companies put a lot of money into developing a drug, they may be biased and push scientists into showing that the clinical trial data works. So they appoint independent researchers to evaluate the drug. On the face of it this is exactly what Gilead did. However, a little more detective work shows that most of the "independent" scientists who did the study actually receive grant funding from Gilead for other research that they conduct. Academics who are reliant on grant funding for their livelihoods are not likely to analyse the data from their main funding in as unbiased a fashion as they should. Coupled with this, it is always possible to use some statistical wizardry to show you the results you want to see.

You are probably wondering how any company could be so stupid, surely manufacturing or manipulating data in this way is fraud and they will be found out when the drug doesn't work. To that I would respond with the following facts. The share price of Gilead rose from 63 USD in January 2020 to a peak of just under 84 USD in April 2020 when remdesivir started being used. The share price has since sunk to about 60-65 USD again. This decrease in share price has no doubt been down to Remdesivir, the sales of which account for 25% of Gilead´s profits (2.8 billion USD in 2020), being slated by the medical community. The world health organisation (WHO) has said there is no benefit to using the drug, but it is still used widely because there is simply no other treatment and there are no major negative side effects to the drug. That's right, doctors continue to administer an expensive drug (each treatment costs the hospital 2 340.00 USD per patient and 4.65 USD to manufacture) that all the evidence shows has no benefit to the patient. They do this because giving a drug feels better than giving nothing. Doctors treating patients with severe SARS-cov-2 are going through extremely difficult times. The feeling of helplessness must be overwhelming as there is nothing they can do to alleviate their patient's suffering. To have seen as much pain and death as they have in this pandemic, I do not begrudge them prescribing and administering a drug that at one point was believed to work and that everyone agrees does not have any bad side effects. If you have nothing to lose you may as well administer the drug. Many doctors are also just following the advice of health boards and politicians, many of whom are lobbied by large pharmaceutical companies like Gilead.

Interestingly, the Congolese government found that Remdesivir was "not as effective as other treatments" in treating ebola and the drug failed clinical trials for the treatment of hepatitis C.

## Hydroxychloroquine

An antimalarial drug used in certain regions around the world, hydroxychloroquine has also been used to treat rheumatoid arthritis, lupus (when the immune system malfunctions and attacks the body) and porphyria (a liver disease that causes chemicals called porphyrins to accumulate in the body). One thing all these diseases have in common is that none of them are caused by viruses. One interesting thing about this and most other anti-malarial drugs is that no one really knows how they work. The exact mechanisms by which drugs work is not always known, once a drug has been shown to be effective at treating a disease the money to research how it actually does so normally dries up. Most people and companies are just happy to have a working medicine and are not always willing to research how it is actually helping us. That being said, we do know a little more about hydroxychloroquine and how it treats autoimmune diseases like lupus. The drug will actually enter and accumulate inside several immune cells, including macrophages and antigen-presenting cells. Once inside they damage these cells and prevent them from working properly. They do this by increasing the pH inside the cells, making them less acidic than they need to be to work. Remember these are the cells that will break apart virions either to completely destroy them (macrophages) or to then carry the different parts of the virion to the memory B-cells and T-cells to trigger a targeted immune response (antigen presenting cells).

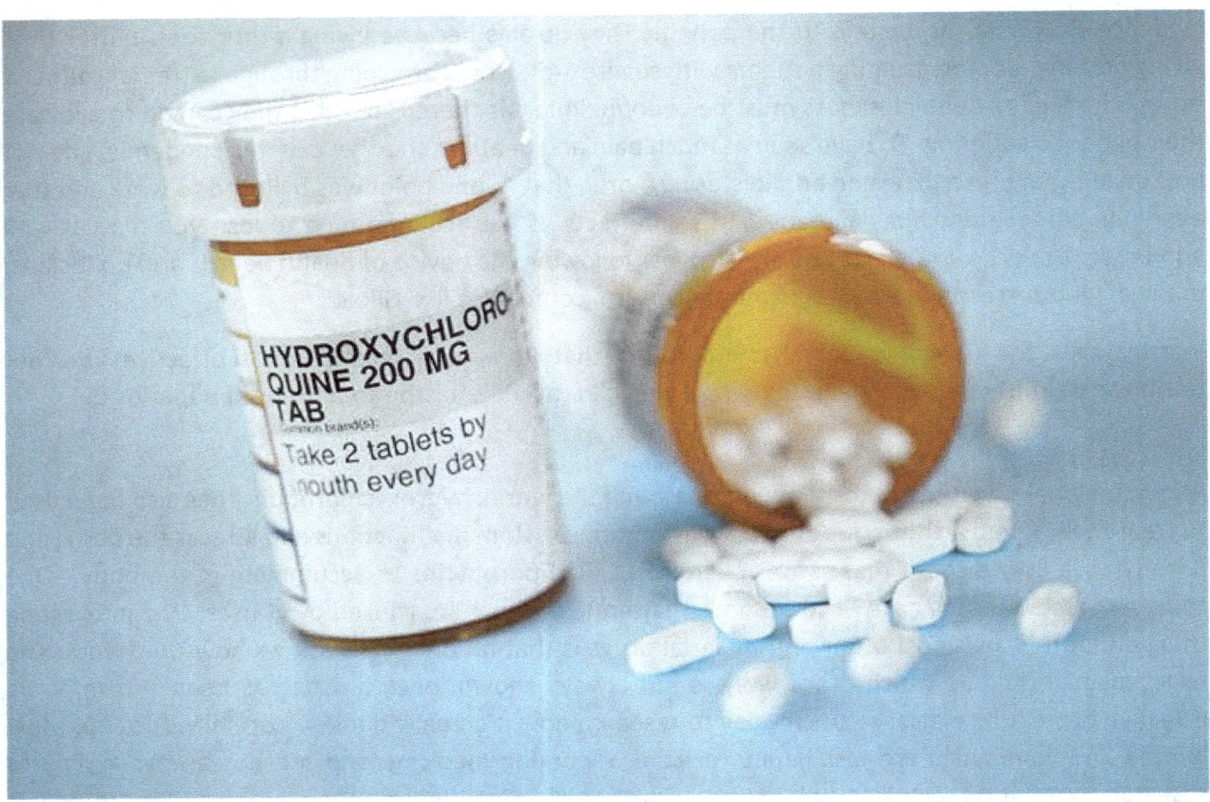

You might be thinking that this would lower inflammation and lessen or stop any serious symptoms of SARS-cov-2. Unfortunately, not. This drug has been shown to be completely ineffective in fighting the disease and can actually make things worse. How? Well the drug has no effect on neutrophils, those cells in the immune system that show up and release toxins to kill nearby cells. Also, by preventing macrophages from working, none of the virions or infected cells can be "eaten". By lowering the immune response, the virus can also spread to other cells in your body more quickly than if you didn't take the drug.

Despite this there have been several high profile public figures that have used the drug routinely, including the former president of the U.S.A., Donald Trump (who got SARS-cov-2 which should prove the hydroxychloroquine doesn't work). You may also be interested to know that "Shi Zheng-Li", a professor at the Wuhan Institute of Virology, who published the first scientific paper on covid-19 and was researching the RaTG13 strain of the coronavirus actually applied for a patent to use chloroquine (closely related to hydroxychloroquine) and remdesivir to treat SARS-cov-2 in China.

## Drinking bleaches and disinfectant

So bleaches and disinfectants are very effective at killing the virus on surfaces, as a result of this the then president of the united states publicly proposed drinking or injecting bleaches or disinfectants as a method of treating SARS-cov-2. This is not a great idea for several reasons. First, the virus is mainly infecting cells in the lungs. When we drink things they go into our stomachs not our lungs, so drinking it definitely won't work. Secondly, bleaches and disinfectants are toxic and corrosive and can cause serious damage and even death. The president made his claims in April of 2020 and since then there have been months of articles and reports debunking this myth. Despite that however, you can still go on amazon today and buy bleach as a "miracle cure" for SARS-cov-2; and people continue to buy it. Yes, despite how dangerous this is people are self-medicating with bleach and the sellers who market it as "Miracle Medical Solution (MMS)", also claim it is effective against cancer, HIV, autism and malaria.

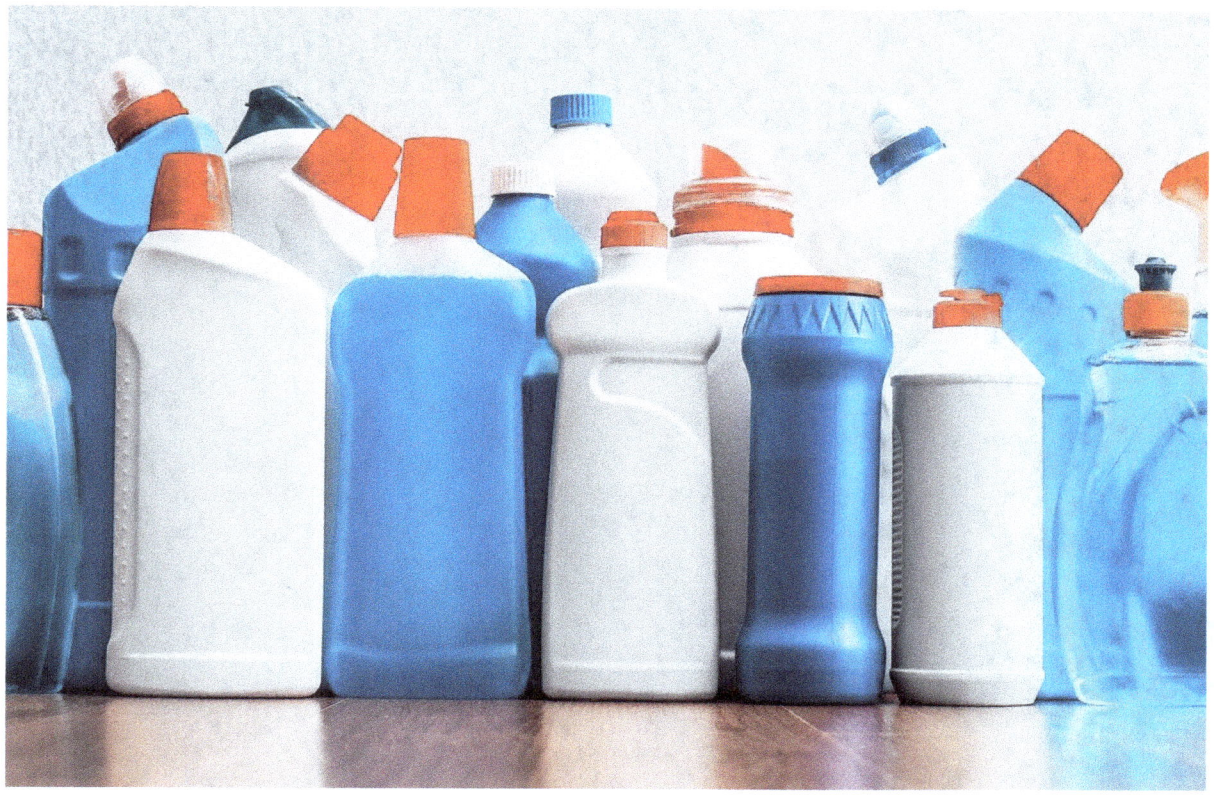

For the record there is no scientific data showing that injecting or drinking bleach is a cure for SARS-cov-2, cancer, HIV, autism, malaria or anything at all. Please do not do drink bleach, it literally has a warning sticker on it saying it needs to be kept away from children so they don't drink it. That's why bottles of bleach have those child-proof caps.

## Getting sunlight into people to destroy the virus

As he made the claim that injecting disinfectant could cure the virus, Donald Trump also suggested putting sunlight into the body to kill the virus. For starters, this doesn't work; but it is not as stupid or as farfetched an idea as the disinfectant. Light is used in medicine quite a lot, and can kill the virus.

There has been quite a lot of research into and development of light based medical treatments. Most people are aware of the fact that sunlight is needed for the skin to produce vitamin D, but there are advanced treatments that utilise light, such as photodynamic therapy. Any child that has ever had a torch will have almost certainly put in in their mouths and seen their cheeks go red. Likewise, if you hold a torch against your hand you will see some light coming through, and it will be red. This is because white light is comprised of light of different wavelengths. The different wavelengths of light have different colours, and red light can penetrate further through the skin and body than any other wavelength of light. Chemists have developed special chemicals (porphyrin photosensitizers) that are completely inactive normally, but will react with red light and become toxic. These can be injected into people and then red light shone on a tumour within the body, the chemical in that area become toxic and the cancer cells are killed.

Sunlight is also known to kill viruses. In this instance the main way it does so uses a different wavelength of light. Ultraviolet (UV) light has a wavelength too small for the human eye to see, although interestingly some animals such as bees do see UV light and some flowers have UV pigments to attract bees that we cannot see. If you ever have the time I would recommend looking up pictures of flowers under UV light as they are quite spectacular. UV light is antiviral because it has the unique ability to create "oxygen radicals". Oxygen radicals are every bit as cool and interesting as they sound. Basically what happens is that UV light will collide with oxygen atoms and knock one of the atom's electrons completely out of the atomic structure. This makes the oxygen extremely reactive. In fact, radicals are so reactive that they are impossible to detect as they react with anything nearby too fast for scientists to detect them. The oxygen radicals generated by UV light will, over time, react with and break apart anything that is exposed to them by chemically damaging the RNA and proteins that make up the virus.

The wavelength of radiation required to make oxygen radicals is absorbed by oxygen in the upper atmosphere and the resulting reaction is what creates ozone. Very little of it reaches the earth's surface so this is not the reason that infection numbers go down in the summer. UV light is also mainly absorbed by the skin and does not pass through the body like red light does. As such it is not possible to get UV light into the body where it is needed to kill the virus. As in the case of drinking bleach, there is no point giving a treatment that kills the virus that will also kill the patient. Over exposure to UV light will just burn the skin and eventually lead to skin cancer.

## Monoclonal antibody treatments

Trials of monoclonal antibodies to treat SARS-cov-2 started in earnest in November of 2020. Their use is currently being investigated in serious cases or those who are in high risk groups who get sick. In essence, this treatment involves taking antibodies from people who have fought off the infection and injecting them into those who are sick. In the section on antibodies, I discussed how B-cells produce antibodies and that naturally, lots of different antibodies capable of binding to the spike protein of cov-19 are produced by a health immune system. If we were to take all of these from one person and use them then this would be termed a "polyclonal antibody treatment". In reality we need to mass produce the best antibody. We do this by taking the DNA sequence for the antibody that experiments show works best and insert this into yeast or bacteria. These are then grown on mass, harvested and the single type of antibody produced is injected into the patient. The difference between polyclonal and monoclonal is the number of different types of antibody used. Whilst monoclonal only uses one type of antibody, there are a large number of copies (clones) of that antibody given in the treatment. I will at this point refrain from comparing these antibodies to storm troopers in "the clone wars", as Star Wars references are not really my thing.

At the time of writing, the monoclonal antibody drugs being tested are called Bamlanivimab, casirivimab and imdevimab. The "-mab" suffix denotes that these are monoclonal antibodies. Currently, the drugs have not been trialled in enough people to be sure that they work. Although the results are promising these drugs are unlikely to be widely available any time soon and it is unlikely that they will be the magic bullet that cures all SARS-cov-2 cases. As with all the other available treatments, mutations in the virus can allow it to evade treatment by this method.

## Vaccines

The first vaccines for cov-19 were rolled out in December of 2020. There are a variety of different vaccines made by different companies coming onto the market. But what exactly are vaccines and how do they work? The general principle of a vaccine is quite simple; it is trying to train your immune system how to fight off a virus or bacteria without you actually having an infection. The invention of the first ever vaccine is credited to the English physician Dr Edward Jenner in 1796, to vaccinate against smallpox. Jenner's breakthrough came when he noticed that the number of milkmaids who got smallpox was much lower than that of the rest of the population. He was also aware of the fact that milkmaids tended to get a similar but much less deadly disease called cowpox, from cows. His theory was that having had cowpox, the milkmaids built up an immunity to whatever was causing smallpox (viruses were not discovered until 1892). To test his theory, he devised one of the most dangerous and unethical experiments in human history.

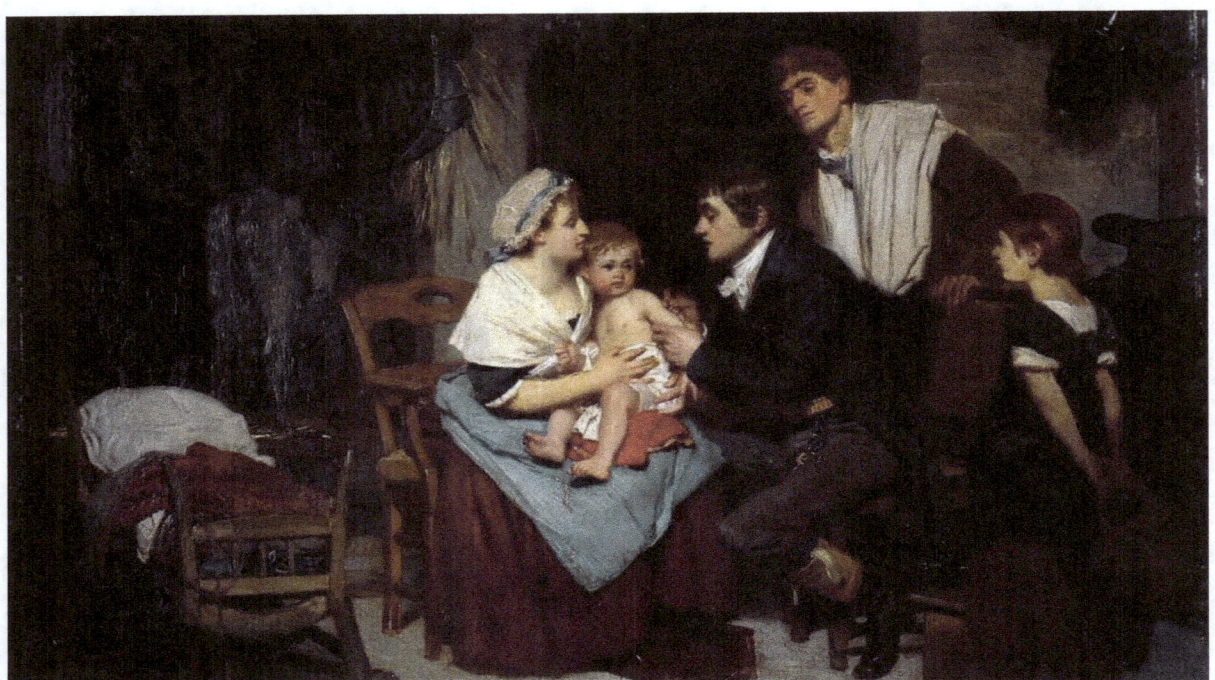

Dr Jenner took the pus from pustules of a milkmaid suffering with cowpox. He then cut the arms of his gardener's 8-year-old son (James Phipps) and smeared the wounds with the pus. This of course led to the boy getting cowpox and becoming mildly ill with the disease. Six weeks later, the experiment was repeated but with pus from a smallpox patient rather than cowpox. James Phipps was exposed to the virus 20 times in total and not once did he become sick with smallpox, leading to him being declared immune. The cowpox virus' Latin name is *Variolae vaccinae* and has given us the words "vaccine" and "vaccination". Because the smallpox and cowpox spike proteins are so similar, the immune system of anyone who got cowpox had antibodies and T-cells that could be triggered to quickly fight off the smallpox virus, thinking it was cowpox.

Whilst Dr Jenner is credited for having invented vaccinations; and his published article of these experiments is the first published account of a vaccine on record; this is not the first instance of immunising people against diseases. In fact, inoculation, the practice of artificially immunising against infectious diseases, has been performed since before records began. Variolation, in which pus or scabs from people suffering with smallpox would be put onto cuts in the arms of people who were healthy was widely used in China, India and the middle east. In these types of inoculation, the pus contains dead host cells, dead immune cells, antibodies and virions that had been inactivated by the immune system. Variolation only made it to Europe in the 1720s and was more dangerous than vaccinations as full blown smallpox infections could sometimes occur. In these cases, the active form of the virus was in the pus. The main benefit of vaccination over Variolation is that in a vaccine, the immune system is trained using a less dangerous, or completely safe, form of the virus.

The principle behind most conventional vaccine manufacturing is quite simple. To generate a safe form of the virus or to find a way of exposing the immune system to spike proteins that appear on the virus so it can be recognised in the future. One method of doing this is to grow the virus in large quantities and then inactive it or make it less dangerous (attenuated). The trick is to stop the virus from being able to infect host cells and cause an infection whilst retaining its structure so that the immune system can learn to identify and fight it. This is normally done by heat, chemical treatment or radiation. In other vaccines, specific proteins (normally the spike proteins) can be isolated, mass produced and used in the vaccine. Whilst the principle is simple, keeping the virus and/or proteins in the right shape whilst inactivating the virus is very difficult practically and requires lots of work to get right. Attenuated vaccines, in which a less dangerous form of the virus is administered as a vaccine, tend to provide a stronger and more robust immune response. These are developed by culturing (growing) the virus and trying to get it to evolve into a less dangerous form. This can be sped up by different methods such as growing them in cells they are less comfortable in, for example animal cells.

## Booster doses

Why do we sometimes need to get vaccinations for the same disease several times? Vaccine boosters, where the vaccine is given again a set time after the first vaccination is routinely done for some, but not all, viruses. There are a couple of different reasons why this might be done. The purpose of every vaccine is to leave the patient with memory T-cells and memory B-cells to fight off the infection if it should appear again. Unfortunately, these memory B-cells and T-cells are not immortal and can die off eventually. For reasons that we do not understand, the immune cells for different diseases die at different rates. The memory T-cells and B-cells for the same virus that are made from different vaccines may also die at different rates. For example, let's look at the polio vaccine. There are two main polio vaccines, one given orally and one given by injection. The oral vaccines only provide immunity for six months. Even further boosters will only provide immunity for a further six months after each booster. By contrast, the injected polio vaccine is given in 4 doses, three before you are 18 months old and one between the ages of 4-6 years. After this the person is immune for life. Whilst polio has been eradicated from the first world, cases in third world countries actually started to increase in 2019 and 2020 where the injected polio vaccine is too expensive to be widely used and only the oral vaccine is more common.

Flu vaccines are given annually, not necessarily because the B-cells and T-cells specific to the flu virus die off, but because the flu virus mutates to rapidly that the vaccines are no longer effective. The flu virus has two spike proteins that are constantly mutating and every year a panel of experts look at global trends in the mutations to determine (make an educated guess) which mutations are most likely to spread that year and develop vaccines for those specific strains of the virus. In fact, the annual flu vaccine is a mixture of around 5 vaccines for the 5 most likely viruses that are going around that year. The rate of mutation of a virus can render vaccines and the immunity they provide redundant after a period of time. The long term effectiveness of covid-19 vaccinations is unknown since the virus and the vaccines are so new.

## How do we know if vaccines are safe and work before giving them to people?

Pre-clinical trial tests are always conducted within laboratories to determine if a vaccine is dangerous or has any chance of working. Usually this involves taking living cells and exposing them to the potential vaccine and seeing whether or not they die. This needs to be done with human cells from different organs, such as the liver, lungs, heart, etc. Normally this process alone can take years. Any vaccine candidates that are found to not kill off healthy cells are then tested for their "efficacy", whether they actually work on cell models. This process involves taking healthy cells and exposing them to the vaccine to see if they start to produce spike proteins. Any candidates that pass the first two series of tests will be taken to animal trials. Now this can be controversial as many people are against animal testing. But it is necessary to determine if there is some reaction that the vaccine candidates have when in a whole living creature as opposed to just in cells on a petri dish. There are many drugs that are completely safe in cell culture tests but undergo a chemical reaction in one organ that turns them into something very toxic to another organ. Animal models are our best and only method of testing whether this happens with any new vaccine or drug.

Any drug candidate that passes all those tests, which in normal circumstances can take many years, now has to face one final challenge before it starts human trials, "scaling up". Just because it is possible to make a vaccine in a lab does not mean that it is possible to make enough for 8 billion people to each get multiple injections. In fact, sometimes it is just difficult to make enough for proper clinical trials. The art of taking a lab based vaccine preparation protocol and scaling it up for mass production is not an easy skill to master. There is an entire industry devoted to just this task. Many vaccine candidates that work in labs are simply unable to be reproduced on the scale needed for mass production. Sometimes this is down to technical reasons, but sometimes the reasons are financial. A hard fact of life is that if a vaccine costs more to produce than we are able to pay for it, then the vaccines will not get made. However, thankfully there are vaccines on the market that made it over all of these hurdles to human clinical trials. Just getting to this stage in normal drug or vaccine development can take many years and cost tens to hundreds of millions of dollars (USD).

Phase 1 clinical trials are tested on small groups of 20-100 volunteers. These people are meticulously selected to be absolutely healthy. They have no underlying health conditions, are not taking any medication (prescription or otherwise), have no disabilities and have never been involved in trialling another drug. The last thing you want is to halt a trial early thinking that it causes serious side effects because someone has a symptom from another disease or the vaccine reacts with a medication they are currently taking. The purpose of these trials is firstly to determine if the vaccine is safe in humans, just because a vaccine is safe in animals does not always mean it is safe in people. Any potential side effects are monitored and safe and appropriate doses are determined at this stage. Antibody tests of the volunteers' blood are also performed to determine if, when and how many antibodies they are producing, a good indication of if, and how well, the vaccine at that dose is working. If the volunteers don't produce any antibodies, get sick or have serious side effects; then the trial ends here.

Phase 2 clinical trials are conducted on several hundred still healthy volunteers. By this point the doses are usually figured out and how common different side effects are can be determined in a larger sample size. At this point it is possible to get a better understanding of how well people's immune systems are responding to the vaccine. By the end of phase 2, it is pretty well established that the vaccines are safe. However, there is no data at this stage as to whether the vaccines actually work.

Phase 3 clinical trials where we get the real data on how well the vaccines work. Here the vaccines are given to thousands of people. A group of volunteers is split in half and one half is given the vaccine whilst the other is given a placebo (essentially just water). For the covid-19 vaccines lots of volunteers were tested and just went about their normal lives. The numbers of each of the two groups (placebo and vaccine) who ended up getting the virus was then compared. If the vaccine works, then the number of people who get SARS-cov-2 will be significantly smaller in the group of people who got the vaccine compared to those who got the placebo. Now the most important word of that last sentence is the word "significantly". In all modern science and statistics where or not the difference between two numbers is "significant" is key.

So what is meant by significance? Imagine you toss a coin 100 times, you would expect that 50 times it would land heads up and 50 times it would land tails facing up. If you actually did this 100 time and it landed heads up 52 times and tails up 48 times you would say this is just down to random chance. In this instance, even though the numbers are not identical you say they are roughly the same and so the difference between them is not "significant". However, if you flipped the coin 100 times and it landed heads up 90 times and tails up 10 times then you might start to say that the coin is weighted or something fishy is going on. Here the difference is significant, our theory that we would get 50 heads and 50 tails is completely wrong. So where do we draw the line? Would 45 heads and 55 tails be significant? What about a 60-40 split? This is where statistics become important. There are a variety of different statistical models that can be used to determine if the difference between two numbers is significant. For the purposes of this book I will not go into detail about the statistics as it is very dry and based on the data from the vaccine trials not necessary. When I discuss the difference in the number of people who got SARS-cov-2 in each vaccine's phase 3 trial data you should be able to get a decent feeling without any statistical analysis.

How does this apply to covid-vaccinations? Imagine we have 10 000 volunteers for our phase 3 clinical trial. A placebo is given to 5 000 and the vaccine given to the other 5 000. If we come back a month later and look at how many people from each group got went on to get SARS-cov-2, if the vaccine doesn't work, we would expect that the number of people who got sick to be the same in both groups. Now they may not be exactly the same, but is the difference between them significant? Ideally no one who got the vaccine would get sick, but I can tell you now (#spoileralert) this was not the case for any of the vaccines. Also things get even more complicated when you delve further into the data. Do those who get the vaccine and get sick mainly come from a specific gender, race, age group, socioeconomic background; do these factors influence the efficacy of the vaccine? By the time you start exploring all these differences (variables) in the data you may not have enough data to say any trend you observe is significant. Taking it back to the coin analogy, if you only flip the coin twice you would expect 1 heads and 1 tails; but wouldn't be surprised to get two heads or two tails in a row. The purpose of Phase 3 clinical trials is usually only to tell us that a vaccine works well enough to merit being rolled out to the general public. However, if the trial is large enough, sometimes trends in different parts of the population can be observed, however lots of data really comes from phase 4 of the clinical trials.

Have you ever taken any medication or been given any vaccine? Congratulations, you have taken part in a phase 4 clinical trial. Thank you for your efforts, give yourself a pat on the back, you should be proud of your contribution to the betterment of the human race. If you have never taken any medicine or refused to be vaccinated… then I am assuming you are an "antivaxer" who has some belief system that opposes western medicine (and the chances of you reading this, or any other, book are very slim). Well guess what. You are also part of the experiment! You are just the control data, no different to anyone on a placebo. We have all taken part, willingly or not, in phase 4 clinical trials for drugs and vaccines throughout our entire lives. Every drug or vaccine that is prescribed or bought is monitored for potential side effects and trends in people who get sick after vaccination and their general data are continuously studied and analysed. This is where the real trends in data, such as if the vaccine is less effective in people with different underlying health conditions (such as obesity or diabetes) who would be excluded from all the other clinical trial phases can be examined. Likewise, the data pool is so large that significant differences between ethnic groups and genders can be determined. All vaccines and drugs remain under constant review until they are no longer used. One of the reasons for this is to make sure they do not cause serious side effects when taken in conjunction with new medicines.

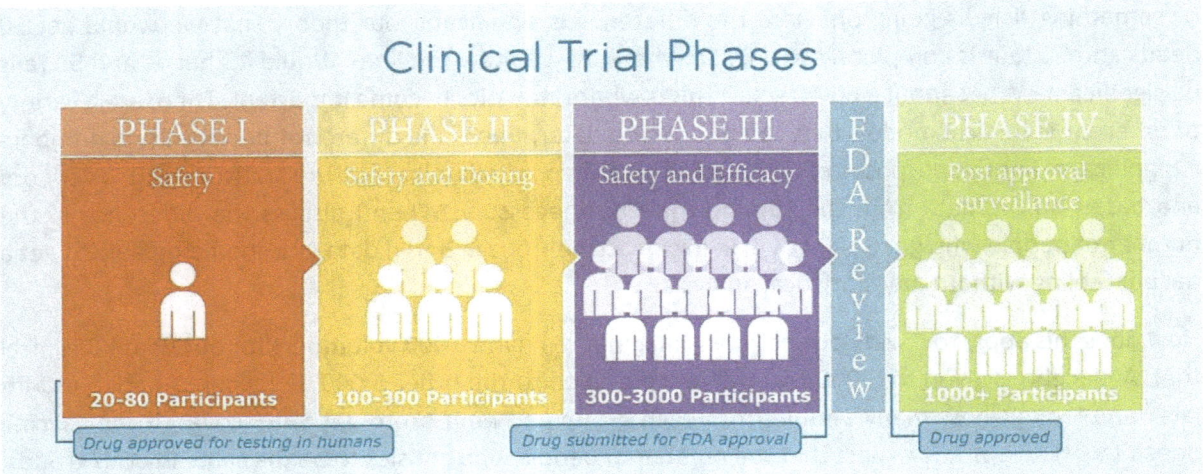

### The current covid 19 vaccines on the market

Several companies have developed vaccines to the cov-19 coronavirus. These work by slightly different methods and I will go through each of them in turn. In principle all these vaccines work by exposing the immune system to the covid-19 spike protein rather than inactive or attenuated forms of the virus.

There have been many myths and conspiracy theories surrounding vaccines in recent years, I will therefore list the ingredients within each of the vaccines and explain what they are and why they are in there. In all vaccinations you are exposing the immune system to a foreign body and triggering an immune response. As such, you can always get "sick" from any vaccine as inflammation is a healthy part of the immune response. However, you will never get as sick as if you had the virus and there is a good chance you will have no "symptoms" or side effects at all.

At the time of writing this book, these are the only vaccines available on the market. Pharmaceutical companies such as Johnson and Johnson, Janssen and Novavax also have vaccines currently going through trials but will not be discussed here as they are not currently on the market.

### The Pfizer-BioNTech vaccine

This is a new type of vaccination which works by a different method to previous vaccines. Most conventional vaccines contain the spike proteins of the virus they are training your immune system to fight. The BioNTech vaccine contains RNA with a sequence that codes for the coronavirus spike protein. This RNA gets inside your cells and starts to be converted into spike proteins. Your immune system will then detect these spike proteins and start to develop an immune response. RNA vaccines are completely new and quite interesting. Before I discuss some of the expected benefits of this method of vaccination, I should make it clear that your cells being hijacked to make viral proteins does sound a lot like having a viral infection. However, because only the spike protein is being made, no virions are being produced, so you will not be contagious and the virus cannot spread through your body.

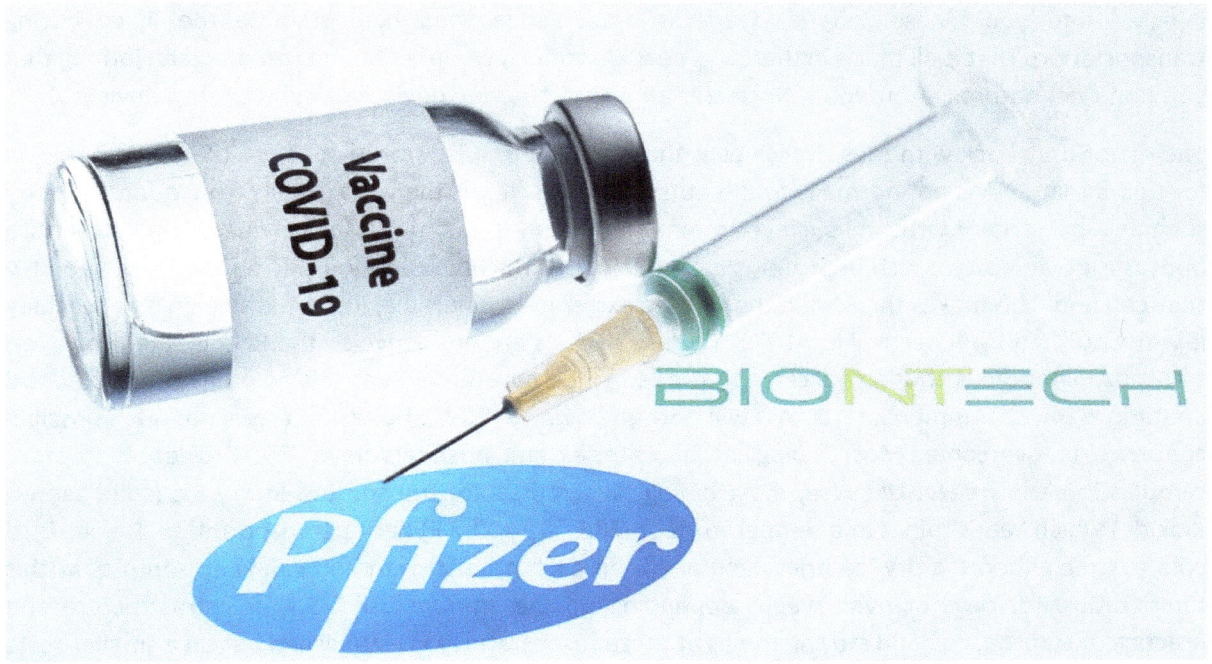

RNA based vaccinations have several benefits over conventional vaccines. Mass producing proteins for vaccinations is a very difficult process and requires lots of large and expensive equipment to manufacture on the scale needed to inoculate large numbers of people. RNA vaccines by contrast are much simpler and easier to make and scale up, since the spike proteins are being made by the patient. If the virus mutates, it is much easier to change the RNA sequence in the vaccine to mirror this mutation and develop vaccines against new viral strains. There is no evidence, or reason to believe, that this type of vaccine has any biological advantage over traditional vaccines; the benefits are all in the manufacturing processes.

Pfizer BioNTech vaccines are meant to be administered by two injections in the arm three weeks apart. By doing so, the second injection is given when the number of antibodies, B-cells and T-cells formed against the virus is at its highest, so re-administering the vaccine will increase the likelihood and number of memory T-cells and B-cells created, which might increase the long term immunity provided by the vaccination.

The Pfizer-BioNTech vaccine contains the following ingredients:

mRNA, lipids ((4-hydroxybutyl)azanediyl)bis(hexane-6,1-diyl)bis(2-hexyldecanoate), 2 [(polyethylene glycol)-2000]-N,N-ditetradecylacetamide, 1,2-Distearoyl-sn-glycero-3-phosphocholine, and cholesterol), potassium chloride, monobasic potassium phosphate, sodium chloride, dibasic sodium phosphate dihydrate and sucrose.

So the first ingredient is obviously the RNA sequence needed to make the spike protein. The lipids are the lipid bilayers like those the viral envelope and your cells are made out of. They are used here to create a parcel in which the RNA is kept safe so it doesn't get destroyed before entering your cells. These lipids are made out of 4-hydroxybutyl)azanediyl)bis(hexane-6,1-diyl)bis(2-hexyldecanoate) and 1,2-Distearoyl-sn-glycero-3-phosphocholine. They also contain cholesterol which makes the lipids more rigid, as it does in your body. Polyethylene glycol is a common chemical even found in some foods, it is a dispersant and stops the lipids from sticking to each other. Every other ingredient is a salt, the concentrations and ratios of which are made to mimic human blood. That way the pH and salinity of the vaccine mimic those in your body and the lipids will not burst or collapse as soon as they are injected into you. These salts also act as preservatives and help stabilise the lipids during transportation. That is all that's in there. Some RNA, some fat, some salt and some sugar. Nothing that you don't get naturally from food. No secret antennas, tracking devices or mind control devices.

The major drawback with these vaccines is that they need to be stored at -70 °C (-94 F). The reason for this is that RNA is not normally found outside of cells. If it is then it is usually from a foreign body such as a bacteria or virus. As such your immune system is very defensive against RNA. Your entire body, inside and out, is rich in proteins called RNAses, which will very quickly destroy any free RNA they can find. This makes the RNA in the vaccine extremely vulnerable, just breathing on it or touching it with your hand will destroy it. At -70 °C these RNAses are not active so the RNA is safe. However, transporting and distributing vaccines that need to be constantly kept this cold has many practical limitations, most commercial freezers will only go down to -20 °C. However, this is not an impossible challenge to overcome. Most biological laboratories and hospitals have -80 °C freezers to store samples in deep freeze. Likewise, most biological samples are transported in dry ice (solid carbon dioxide) which keeps things at a temperature of -78.5 °C (-109.2 F) during transportation. Dry ice is so cold that neighbouring dry ice bricks actually keep each other frozen and can keep samples at this temperature for days or even weeks depending on the amount used. So the infrastructure and practice of transporting and storing things at these temperatures is established but on a smaller scale than what is required for vaccinating everyone who would need vaccinated. These vaccines need to be defrosted just before use which can take several hours. Once defrosted they cannot be re-frozen so must be used or discarded straight after defrosting. The dangers of re-freezing are that the RNA may have been destroyed when thawed and repeated freezing and thawing can damage the lipids.

## Pfizer BioNTech Phase 3 clinical trial data

The data from the phase 3 clinical trials of the Pfizer-BioNTech vaccine can be summarised into the following key facts. Over 43 000 volunteers were part of this study, of this number over 20 000 would have been given the vaccine and over 20 000 were given a placebo. The exact number in each group is never the same as some people will pull out of the study part of the way through or may need to be excluded. Remember these are real people living normal lives, things come up that prevent them from being able to continue in a study such as having to attend funerals, work commitments, etc. Sometimes people's data is removed from the study but only when there is an appropriate reason to do so. For example, if a volunteer contracts SARS-cov-2 on their way home from their first injection, before the vaccine has had time to work, then their data can be removed by those analysing the vaccine. Every person's data that is excluded has to be disclosed in full with an explanation and justification of why it has been excluded. Failure to do this is fraud, the governing bodies that determine whether a drug is safe are extremely strict about these things, as they should be. In the Pfizer BioNTech trial, of the over 20 000 people who were vaccinated, only 8 people went on to get SARS-cov-2, compared to 162 in the placebo group. You don't need to be a statistician to tell that this is quite a significant difference. From this data it is pretty clear that the vaccine is doing some good.

But 8 people still got sick didn't they? Despite having had the vaccine. Very few vaccines are 100% effective so this is not surprising. Everyone's immune systems are different and some people will just not generate an adequate immune response even after vaccination. For most vaccines, even though these people can still get sick the number of people getting severe infections usually decreases as a result of vaccination. Whether or not these vaccines will reduce or even eliminate the number of severe SARS-cov-2 cases will only be determined for certain by analysis in the phase 4 clinical data which does not exist yet. Any volunteers who got infections within 28 days of their first injection were excluded from the study and the data was recorded for two months after the first injection. In other words, all the people who got sick and their data was included in the trial got infected more than 4 weeks but less than 8 weeks after the first injection. It is not known if the vaccine provides immunity for more than a couple of months. Pfizer claims that the vaccine starts to offer some protection 10 days after the first infection but has no data for whether the first jab alone provides protection without the second jab after 21 days, they simply didn't test that. In other words, nobody knows if only one injection is enough to provide you with immunity, all test subjects were given the booster dose.

## The Moderna vaccine

A competing RNA based vaccine has also been developed by Moderna. In principle, this is the same as the Pfizer-BioNTech vaccine. The only difference between them is the chemical make-up of the lipid bilayer that envelopes the RNA. Since this is different, the chemicals used to stabilise it are also different. The Moderna vaccine is more stable and resistant to RNAses than the Pfizer-BioNTech vaccine so can be stored and transported at -20 °C, which makes it better suited for widespread use. Since the lipids are chemically different, it is expected that the rate and amount of RNA that they provide to host cells will differ. This may result in one vaccine infecting more host cells than the other. It is not known whether this actually happens or if this means one type of vaccine is better than the other, it is too early to tell. This vaccine is injected into the muscle and a booster is then given 1 month afterwards.

The Moderna vaccine contains:

Messenger ribonucleic acid (mRNA), lipids (SM-102 (heptadecan-9-yl 8-((2-hydroxyethyl) (6-oxo-6-(undecyloxy) hexyl) amino) octanoate), polyethylene glycol [PEG] 2000 dimyristoyl glycerol [DMG], cholesterol, and 1,2-distearoyl-sn-glycero-3-phosphocholine [DSPC]), tromethamine, tromethamine hydrochloride, acetic acid, sodium acetate and sucrose.

SM-102 (heptadecan-9-yl 8-((2-hydroxyethyl) (6-oxo-6-(undecyloxy) hexyl) amino) octanoate), is a molecule that has been synthesised and patented by Moderna, but is still just a fatty acid that makes a lipid bilayer. As an aside, lots of chemicals that have been developed by companies have names like SM-102, these are normally just acronyms for something like "secret molecule 102". This often leads to some conspiracy theorists saying there is something fishy going on, but it is literally just a filing system for new molecules that a company wants to develop and patent. In this case the polyethylene glycol dispersant has been chemically bonded to DMG which is part of the lipid layer. With the cholesterol and DSPC, these components all form the lipids. The tromethamine, tromethamine hydrochloride, acetic acid, sodium acetate and sucrose are salts and sugar to mimic the pH inside your body and stabilise the lipids.

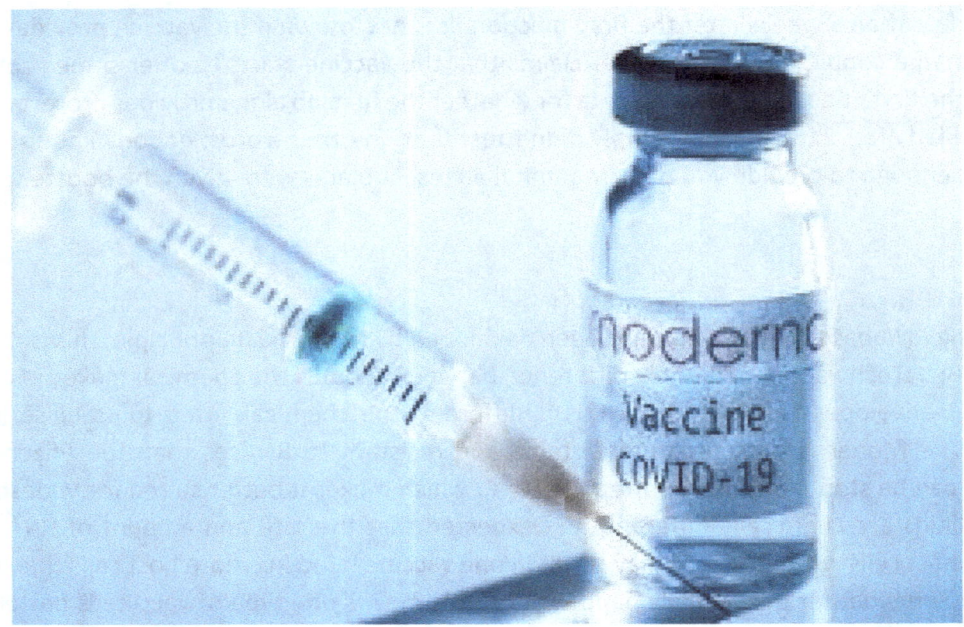

Depending on where you live, some vaccines are approved and some are not. In America the Pfizer and Moderna vaccines are the only two available, and they have been approved for "emergency use". What that means is that there is sufficient evidence the vaccines don't do any harm and that the situation is sufficiently bad that they are willing to let the vaccine be rolled out with less evidence than normal that it works. In other words, this is a life threatening pandemic killing millions of people worldwide, we don't know if these vaccines work but we are convinced they won't do you any harm, so let´s give it a try.

## Moderna vaccine phase 3 clinical trial data

In the Moderna study, 30 420 people volunteered for testing. Of these 15 210 were given the vaccine and 15 210 given a placebo. 4% of participants dropped out of the study before the second dose was administered. In the placebo group, 185 people developed SARS-cov-2, compared to just 11 in the vaccinated group. Of those in the placebo group that got sick, 30 cases were severe (required hospitalisation) and one volunteer died. None of the 11 people who got sick in the vaccinated volunteers had severe covid symptoms. More data is needed to say for certain that this vaccine reduces the severity of coronavirus infections. However, like the Pfizer vaccine, you do not need to be a statistician to say that significantly fewer people got sick who were vaccinated than in the placebo group.

## The Oxford-AstraZeneca vaccine

Also known as the "Oxford vaccine" since it was developed at the University of Oxford, this is the first of the more traditional style of vaccine to be developed and marketed. The technical name for this vaccine is ChAdOx1, and the name tells us a lot about what the vaccine contains. This vaccine has taken an adenovirus (a group of viruses that normally cause the common cold) that only normally infects chimpanzees. Scientists have then genetically modified the virus to contain the genetic sequence for the covid-19 spike protein. These modified adenoviruses were then put onto appropriate chimpanzee cells[4] that they infected and they begin to mass produce adenovirus virions that also had covid-19 spike proteins. The virions can then be removed, cleaned and prepared as vaccines.

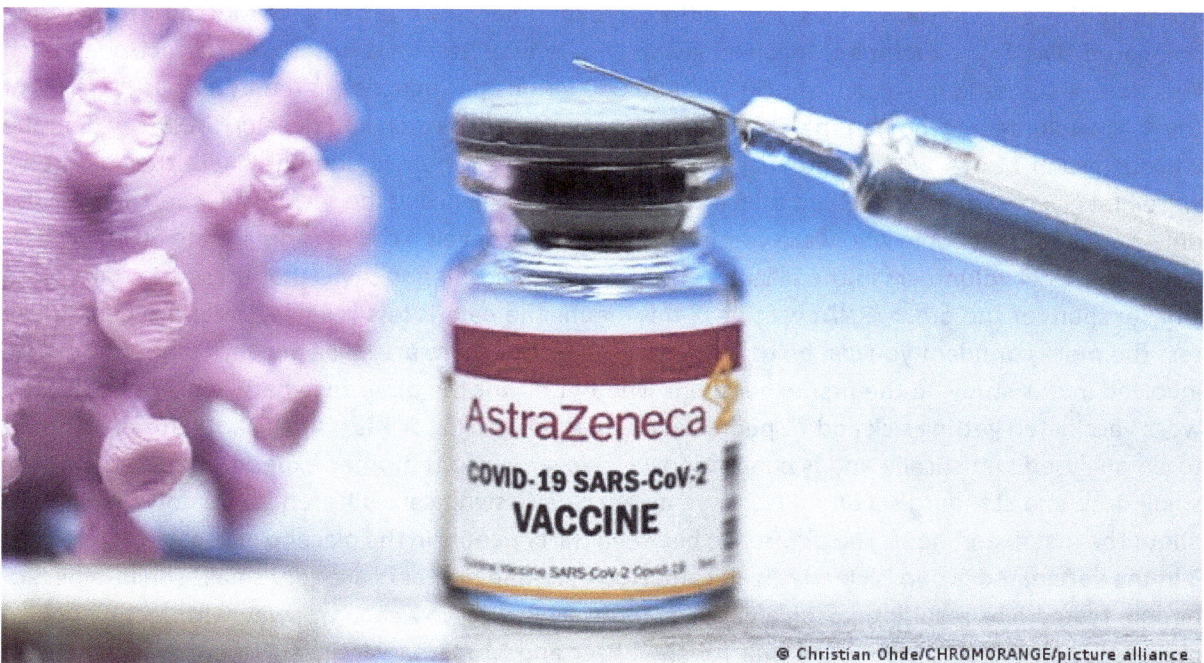

© Christian Ohde/CHROMORANGE/picture alliance

After being injected, these synthetic viruses will travel around your body until the spike proteins find and bind to ACE2 receptors and infect your cells, as the coronavirus would. They then programme your cells to start mass producing the spike proteins. Since none of the other cov-19 virus proteins are present no virions can be made and the infection will not spread, but an immune response will be triggered. Triggering an immune response will always come with the risk of side effects such as inflammation. The AstraZeneca vaccine was originally meant to be administered by two injections three weeks apart. However, the UK government decided that it would administer doses 12 weeks apart. The rational for this is that there are shortages with the vaccines, as the viruses need to be grown and are in high demand; and that their priority is to give as many people as possible the first dose before giving out the second dose. During the clinical trials of this vaccine a smaller patient sample was tested with boosters given 12 weeks rather than 3 weeks after the first injection. Whilst the data appears to show that there is no significant issue with doing this, most scientists are of the opinion that not enough people were included in these tests to draw any concrete conclusions from the data.

The following ingredients are found in this vaccine:

ChAdOx-1, L-Histidine, L-Histidine hydrochloride monohydrate, Magnesium chloride hexahydrate, Polysorbate 80 (E 433), Ethanol, Sucrose, Sodium chloride, Disodium edetate (dihydrate).

All of the ingredients other than the adenovirus (ChAdOx-1) are either salts or sugars that are commonly found in foodstuffs. Again the purpose of these is to stabilise the virus during transportation and storage and to mimic internal pH, etc. Polysorbate 80 (E 433) is an emulsifier, it helps fatty and oily things to dissolve in water, it is commonly used in ice-cream.

---

[4] Harmlessly taken from a chimpanzee. No animals would need to be hurt to develop this vaccine.

## The Oxford-AstraZeneca phase 3 clinical trial data

The data from these trials is a little bit more confusing since they were actually trialling two different doses at the same time. At least two different experiments were being conducted at once and compared. The first experiment involved giving people two "standard doses" of the vaccine at each injection. A standard dose contains 50 000 000 000 virions per injection. When this was done 27 of the 4 440 volunteers who had the ChAdOx1 vaccine went on to catch and develop SARS-cov-2, in the placebo group 71 of 4 445 volunteers got SARS-cov-2. In the other experiment where the volunteers were first given a smaller dose and then a standard dose when giving the second injection; in this case only 3 out of 1367 people who were vaccinated went on to develop covid, compared to 30 volunteers out of the 1374 volunteers in the placebo group. So the first thing to say is that these trials are much smaller than for the other (RNA) vaccines., this means the data is less reliable, the more people you test the more confident you can be that the test works. But there are still a decent number of people involved in this study. In the first experiment whether or not the difference between 27 people who were vaccinated getting sick and 71 people in the placebo getting sick is a significant difference needs to be analysed statistically and is contentious. However, since the other experiment, with an initial small dose and standard second dose, gave a very clearly significant difference, we don't really care about the first experiment. The difference between thirty people in the placebo group getting sick and 3 in the vaccinated group is clearly significant. However, the numbers are very small. The numbers of people tested and resulting positive cases is about as low as you can get away with testing, which makes this data less reliable than that for the Pfizer and Moderna vaccines. Nevertheless, the data presented does indicate that the vaccine works.

The data shows that by giving a smaller first dose and a larger second dose the vaccine works better. Nobody really understands this finding. How or why this is the case is a mystery. There is ongoing research to try to understand why it is the case.

As I was finishing writing this book this vaccine began to make headlines amid fears it triggers blood clotting in some who receive it. Blood clots can cause heart attacks and strokes. The WHO has said that there is no link between the virus and an increased risk of blood clotting. The percentage of those vaccinated experiencing these symptoms is the same as the percentage of the population who have not been vaccinated. However, several governments have taken the decision to temporarily halt the use of the Oxford-AstraZeneca vaccine. It is not known how the vaccine would cause blood clotting, if it does. In time perhaps these fears, like those of using ibuprofen, will disappear and the vaccine will continue to be used. It should be born in mind however that normal vaccine trials have been rushed to fight the pandemic and there may be resulting risks associated with this vaccine from rushing the safety trials.

## How long will the vaccines protect us for?

So all the phase 3 clinical trials for all the vaccines show that they have some beneficial impact in the two months following the injections. But how long will they provide immunity for? So because all these vaccines are so new there is simply no data for how long they provide immunity for. There are two factors that affect how long a vaccine provides immunity for, how long your immune system "remembers" its training (how long your memory B-cells and T-cells survive) and how quickly the virus mutates.

A lot of the general public regard any vaccine as a silver bullet and that once everyone (or enough people) have had their injections we can go back to living our lives like we used to in 2018. Unfortunately, this will almost certainly not be the case. Even with the entire population inoculated the virus can still spread. Vaccines don't stop the virus from infecting people and you can still get sick after being vaccinated. Your immune system is just trained to fight off the viral infection so you get less sick and usually get better faster. The virus will continue to spread and, importantly, mutate. In the last 18 months this virus has evolved to be able to infect bats, people, minks and even tigers. It is mutating very quickly and will evolve in such a way that our immune systems will no longer recognise them, rendering the current vaccines useless. This has already happened in South Africa where new strains of the virus (with N501Y and E404K mutations) spread faster than the original variant, currently accounting for 90% of all South African cases. The E404K mutation has means that this variant is already resistant to the Oxford-AstraZeneca vaccine. As a result, the South African authorities have "paused" their rollout of the Oxford-AstraZeneca vaccine as of February of 2021.

The uncomfortable truth is that this virus is mutating so quickly, that by the time a vaccine is developed and becomes widespread the coronavirus has mutated to avoid it. This is largely reminiscent of the influenza (flu) virus, for which new vaccines need to be developed every 6 months. Unfortunately, since this is a new virus, we do not have the wealth of knowledge needed to predict which strains are going to be most prevalent like we do with the flu, so cannot "predict" which variations to prepare vaccines for. It may take many years for us to get to that point.

There is good news though. Whilst the rapid mutation rate of the virus makes vaccination difficult, it does have a positive aspect. Viruses evolve to become less deadly. There may be a few hiccups along the road, with a few more deadly strains cropping up from time to time, but in general there is an evolution drive for the virus to not cause you any harm. Imagine that three new variants of the virus evolve, the first is extremely deadly, the second makes the host sick but does not kill them, and the third variant causes absolutely no symptoms. Now the first variant evolves within a host and kills them. If the virus kills its host, it is trapped in that body, unable to infect more people. Meanwhile the second variant evolves in a different host. This person feels sick so stays at home in bed, binging on television and avoiding other people, this variant will be able to spread more than the first variant, infecting a few new people. It can spread to others in the house or when the host drags themselves to the shop for groceries but not as much as the third variant. The final strain of the virus mutates in a host who is completely asymptomatic. They have no idea they are sick and go on with their daily lives, meeting with friends and family, going to work, socialising, spreading the virus the entire time. This variant can infect more people than the other, more dangerous, variants. Over time the less severe viral strains will become more widespread, all the time acting kind of like vaccines, training our immune systems how to fight off future infections. Given enough time this virus will go away completely by itself, there may be some symptoms, such as coughing, that help the virus to get between different hosts that will be beneficial for the virus to cause. But more severe cases will decrease as a result of evolution. Now this can take some time, but the faster the virus mutates, the more likely it is to hit upon a new variant that is less dangerous but more transmissible. The more a virus mutates the more likely we are to get to that strain.

Another positive from this pandemic is that these new RNA vaccines work. These can be mass produced in a couple of weeks and changing the RNA sequence to mimic any mutations in the spike protein should be very quick and easy. So if new variants arise it should be much quicker to develop vaccines against them using this new technology. It is entirely possible that we may just need to get regular vaccinations for the newest variants of the coronavirus for many years or decades to come, like we do with the flu.

## Controversy surrounding vaccines

Those who do not "believe" in vaccines are commonly called "anti-vaxxers". Now there is an overwhelming amount of evidence proving that vaccines work. Too much to possibly print in one book. If anyone reading this book is not convinced that vaccines work, just cast your mind back to the last time you saw or heard about someone getting smallpox. The fact is that nobody, not one single person, has died of smallpox since 1977 should prove that vaccines work. Smallpox killed an estimated 300 000 000 people worldwide between 1900 and 1977. To go from that, to not a single person dying from smallpox is an incredible achievement and as concrete evidence of anything, ever. It is not possible to prove anything works more than it has been proven that the smallpox vaccine works.

A small proportion of the population are conspiracy theorists who believe that the vaccines contain mind control chemicals, chemicals that will sterilise them, make them vote a certain way or even turn them into homosexuals. I personally question whether any of them actually believe what they are saying. Most of them are just resorting to sensationalism in order to get views and subscribers on their social media accounts. Whether this is for financial gain or because they want the attention, I think there are instances of both. Personally I also believe the media are also largely responsible for an upsurge in conspiracy theorists. The media often resort to hyperbole in order to gain traction and interest on a particular story, probably because the traditional mainstream media market is in decline. This normalises extreme opinions that others copy and in some instances exaggerate in order to captivate an audience. Let´s face it, as interesting as I might find RNA vaccine technology, most people are more likely to read or watch a conspiracy theory video about vaccines allowing the government to control their minds than read about how these vaccines actually work.

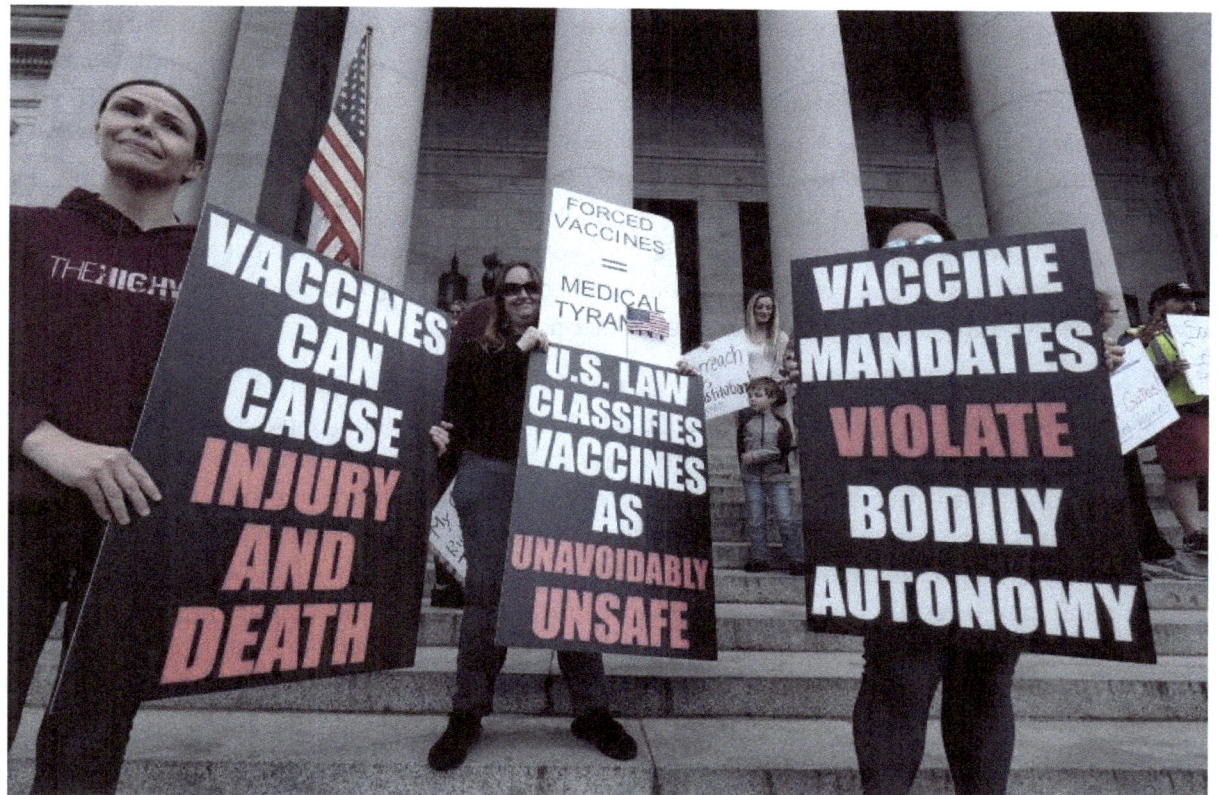

A large proportion of antivaxxers do not, however, have faith based issues in the efficacy of vaccines, nor are they conspiracy theorists; rather they are concerned about the safety of vaccines. Now for this is there are some previous historical examples of vaccines being dangerous, but far more often than not they are completely safe. Part of me including the section on clinical trials above is to show the reader the amount of safety and testing required before a vaccine is given to the general public. Perhaps the best example of safety concerns around vaccines come from the Measles, Mumps and Rubella (MMR) vaccine being linked to autism. In 1998, Andrew Wakefield published a scientific paper showing that 12 children developed autism very shortly after receiving MMR vaccines, and concluded that the vaccines had caused autism. This led to a 20% reduction in vaccinations across the UK. It was later found that Wakefield had received money from families who then went on to try and sue the companies that make the MMR vaccine. The whole thing was a massive case of fraud and Wakefield was struck off of the medical register. By fraud, it was found that Wakefield literally made up and changed the numbers in his paper to show that MMR vaccines caused autism when they categorically do not. This one instance of fraud lead to hundreds of thousands of children not being vaccinated which put their health at risk and created a link between vaccines in general and autism that is completely untrue. There has never been any link between autism and any vaccine. Despite this, the view that there is a link is still held by many. I would urge restraint amongst antivaxxers as every time someone spreads this theory they put children's lives at risk through them potentially not being vaccinated.

So have there ever been cases of vaccines that are dangerous? All vaccines trigger an immune response so there is always a risk of side effects. However, if these side effects are more dangerous than getting the disease, the vaccine would not be used. That being said, there have been several instances of very costly mistakes. The Cutter incident of 1955 is probably one of the most well-known examples of this. In this incident, pharmaceutical company "Cutter" were manufacturing a polio vaccine by inactivating the polio virus. In one batch however, the virus was not inactivated and the live virus was injected into those being inoculated. In total over 250 people were actively given polio.

As a result, many new mandatory safety checks were introduced. The Cutter incident was in itself not a result of the vaccine being dangerous but human negligence and mistakes in the vaccine manufacturing. All recorded incidents with vaccines in history have been as a result of issues (such as contamination) during manufacturing. There has never been any scientifically proven link between any vaccine and any serious health conditions. The worst thing a properly made vaccine will do is make you a little sick. The exception to this is when people have allergic reactions to any of the other components inside the vaccine. If you have allergies, you should always check what is inside a vaccine before getting it. It is a legal requirement that all vaccines and drugs contain and publish a list of ingredients so you can check online before being vaccinated.

There is always debate about the cost of medicines. To get any drug or vaccine to market takes on average 12-18 years and costs on average 2 000 000 000 USD. Considering a patent will last 20 years, that means a pharmaceutical company may have as little as 2 years to recover the cost of developing the drug before copies are made and sold. On top of this they must also cover the costs of any other medicines they tried to develop that fail at any of the stages above. Considering on average only 1 in every 2 000 drug candidates makes it to market, there is usually quite a lot of money to recover. They also have no idea when they will actually be able to release another drug and if a competitor will develop something before them. Just because the final vaccine costs 5 USD to manufacture does not mean it is financially viable to sell it 10 USD. I´m not saying that the costs of some drugs is always justified, but thought I would put some of the numbers involved into context.

# Trends in the SARS-cov-2 cases

## Seasonal trends

There have been several noticeable trends in the number of coronavirus cases over time. The first is that there are more cases during the winter months than during the summer. This is a trend that is observed in all diseases that spread from person to person. There are several theories as to why this happens, but the most widely accepted one is that it is a result of changes in human behaviour. In the summer, when it is warm, people are more likely to spend time outdoors and farther apart from each other. In the colder winter months, people are more likely to stay indoors where we inevitably come into closer contact with each other and spread more diseases.

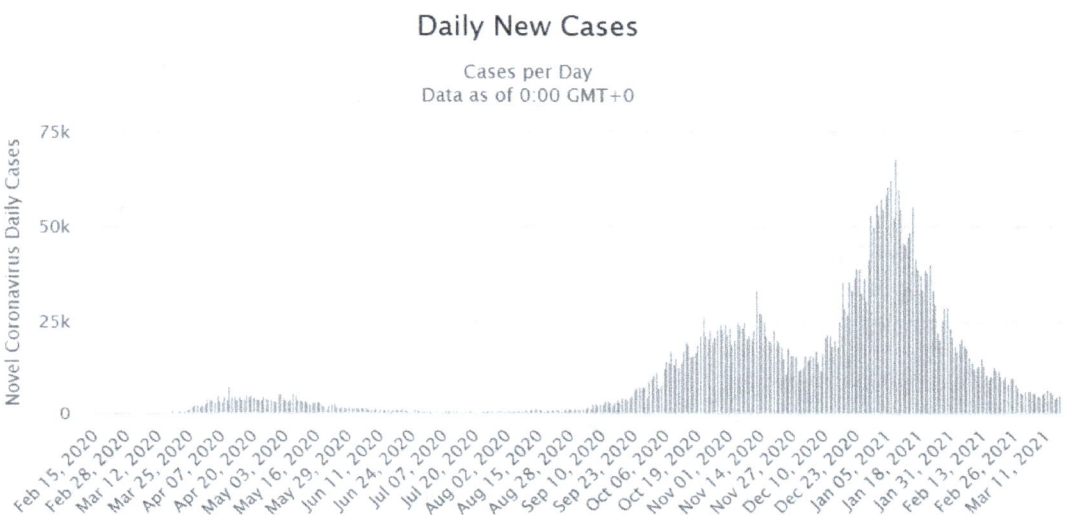

## Age and gender

It is known that anyone of any age can get SARS-cov-2 and die as a result. However, more elderly people are dying than young people. Overall the virus is killing about 4% of people who get it. SARS-cov-2 is killing about 13% of people over the age of 80, 8.6% of those between 70-80, 4% of those between 60-70, 1.25% of those in their 50s and 0.3% of those in their 40s or younger. So there is a clear increase in lethality of the virus amongst older people. But why? As you get older, your immune system generally gets worse.

The number of T-cells you have that are waiting to specialise to fight off a new infection drops drastically, by about 90%, between the ages of 40 and 50. This means when a new infection that your body doesn't recognise comes along, it is harder for the immune system to develop specialised T-cells to fight off that pathogen (virus, bacteria or fungus). Interestingly this is not the only time this happens in your life. The thymus also has a tenfold drop in immune cells during puberty. It seems as though our bodies are designed to learn how to cope with most infections before we develop into adults.

Another factor is that as you get older you have fewer antigen presenting cells, which means fewer spike proteins are presented to B-cells and T-cells. In terms of B-cells, they take longer to develop new antibodies as you get older. This is because B-cells in older people have less of the enzymes that are involved in developing new antibodies. Meaning their chances of hitting on a winning antibody sequence is reduced. Since the T-cells and B-cells are less active, the initial immune response, which is more damaging to healthy cells, is left for longer to fight off the infection alone. As a result, elderly people are more likely to develop more serious symptoms.

Men´s immune responses also typically involve a more aggressive initial, non-specific response than women´s. There are many biological differences between men and women, one of which is a lower number of B-cells and T-cells in men. Yes, "man flu" is in fact a real thing, male immune responses are slower and less specific. This means there is typically more inflammation and therefore worse symptoms in men when they have the same infection as a woman, whether it is covid-19 or not. Another factor is that the different hormones that men and women have also influence immune cells. The differences between men's and women's immune system is in fact very complicated, but there is a trend for men to suffer worse SARS-cov-2 infections than women. In the other recent coronavirus outbreaks (SARS-cov-1 and MERS) about three times more men than women went on to develop serious symptoms.

## Race

There have been many media stories showing that greater proportion of ethnic minorities are contracting SASR-cov-2. There are societal trends that must be taken into consideration when looking at these trends. Immigrants and refugees typically have lower living standards than the general population, often living in overcrowded areas where the virus can spread more easily. Ethnic minorities are typically poorer. Those without savings feel the pressure to go out and work in order to make ends meet which puts them at risk of infection. Being poor increases your risk of contracting SARS-cov-2, and a greater proportion of minority groups are poor; so it is their position within society that puts them at risk.

Are there any biological differences between the races that account for the increased number of cases in ethnic minorities? Before going into this I would like to highlight that race is an extremely controversial topic to write about. Especially biological and genetic differences between races. The data discussed here is not a matter of the authors opinion, nor do the differences make one race "superior". However, like in the case of gender, there are biological differences between different groups in society and we need to understand and appreciate these. Knowledge is power, by understanding the differences in the immune systems of different groups in society we may be able to better protect or treat each other in this and future pandemics.

There are genetic differences between the immune systems of people from different ethnic backgrounds. A recent study found that the immune responses of Europeans is better at dealing with viruses than the immune responses of Africans. The reason found for this is that Europeans mixed more with Neanderthals (a race of cavemen that we *homo sapiens* ended up destroying). As a result, Europeans have Neanderthal DNA in their immune cells that makes them better equipped to fight off viruses than other races. The main result of these genetic differences are that Europeans are better able to regulate inflammation. Africans have more inflammation early on but are less well equipped to reduce inflammation when it becomes dangerous.

## How dangerous is covid-19

Is this virus no worse than the flu? When the virus first emerged there were many people around the world, myself included, who said that the virus was no more dangerous than the flu. This is because, at the time, that "appeared" to be the case. The data that the Chinese government released showed that the death rate from SARS-cov-2 was comparable with the flu virus. Given that some coronavirus outbreaks have indeed been confused for the seasonal flu, most people were not too concerned. It was only when the virus began to spread outside of China that the real death rate (4%) and infectivity (R numbers) became known. For comparison, the flu kills between 300 000 and 650 000 people every year, whereas SARS-cov-2 killed over 2 million people in 2020 alone.

There is the possibility that the Chinese officials made a mistake in the numbers they were releasing, however, to believe this would probably be naïve. It is almost certain that the Chinese authorities lied about the numbers of people dying from SARS-cov-2. They probably did this in an attempt to avoid national embarrassment. However, in trying to cover up the truth and the virus turning into a pandemic, they have only made themselves look even worse. Another unfortunate by-product of the failed cover-up is that it set a fire under the conspiracy theorists and created a culture of mistrust around everything corona related.

This has led to speculation about whether the Chinese continue to tamper with their coronavirus statistics. They report less than 5 000 Chinese have died since the pandemic began. Given the size of the Chinese population and that this was where the outbreak began, these numbers are so low that they are hard to believe. That being said, if any government had the ability to enforce a strict lockdown and prevent the spread of the disease it would probably be the Chinese government. Currently China has some of the strictest lockdown measures in the world, with a mandatory 28-day quarantine in a secure facility for anyone entering the country.

## When will life return to normal?

Looking into a crystal ball and trying to predict anything with coronavirus is difficult. But one thing is for certain, the answer to the question of when life will go "back to normal" is…never. There are lots of reasons for this. One is that society has fundamentally changed as a result of this pandemic and there are many aspects of life in 2018 that people do not want to return too. Countless companies have closed or reduced office spaces, digital companies do not need premises, give your staff a laptop and decent Wi-Fi and they can work from home. Why spend money renting office space you don't need, also the stresses and pollution of commuting are non-existent when working from home. Considering the size of the online economy, a significant section of society will probably start to work from home more often if not all the time.

Perhaps there also needs to be a realisation that life pre-pandemic was not "normal". I am personally opposed to the phrase "the new normal" the truth is that the "new normal" is in fact the "old normal". It is only in the last 100 or so years that we have lived in a world with antibiotics and widespread vaccinations that allow large swathes of the human population to live with fear of death from smallpox, cholera, tuberculosis, dysentery, polio, diphtheria, etc. There are those out there who frown upon modern (sometimes called western) medicine. But its achievements have been staggering. Now, for the first time in living memory, a truly global pandemic has arisen and lives have actually gone back partially to the way they were before all the scientific advances that allowed us to live the way we did. But the way we are living now, with the coronavirus, in fear of getting sick and/or dying; this is the way human kind has lived for all but the last century. That is why I argue that the "new normal" is in fact the "old normal". But its 2021, are we even still supposed to use the word "normal"?

Looking into the future however, we know at some point the virus will mutate to a less dangerous form. It is also highly likely that we will need regular vaccines, like flu vaccines to fend off the newer variants. Anyone who thinks that by the end of 2021 we have all been vaccinated and life will be back to the way it was is, unfortunately, not likely to be right. That being said perhaps the virus will mutate to an extremely transmissible but completely harmless variant tomorrow. There is always a chance.

## The positive impact of the pandemic

Nothing in this world is wholly good or wholly bad. Covid-19 is no exception. Despite all the damage and chaos it has caused, there have been some positives to come out of the pandemic. The first and most widely reported of these is the environmental impact. With travel bans and a drop in commuting because of people working from home, greenhouse gas emissions have dropped significantly. Hopefully societal changes as a result of the pandemic will make more people work from home; a long term reduction in commuters will only be beneficial in slowing global warming. Likewise, with businesses realising that meetings and conferences can be done digitally rather than in person, a reduction in air travel has also been beneficial to the environment.

As lockdowns have been rolled out worldwide, there has been a stark reduction in crime. However, this only applies to certain types of crime, such as theft. It is harder to break into peoples´ homes when they are always there. Other crimes, such as domestic abuse, computer hacking and fraud have either stayed the same or increased during the pandemic.

Some companies have done extremely well out of the pandemic. "Zoom" the video conferencing company was actually started in 2011. Yet it was never able to compete with the likes of "Skype" or "FaceTime". For some reason that nobody really understands, it has completely over-run the market and is now so popular that to "Zoom", is now a verb. Its share price at the start of 2020 was 67 USD, and peaked at 559 USD in October 2020. An article in the financial times has outlined the 100 companies to have done best during the pandemic and sorted them by sector. The obvious trend in all these companies is that they are technology based. It is not surprising that as people are spending more time at home, they are using more technology. Those companies that offer services that offer relief from the realities of self-isolation are doing well.

Companies with net market cap gain of more than $1bn in 2020, by sector. Circle size shows market cap added YTD*, top 100 highlighted, top 25 labelled

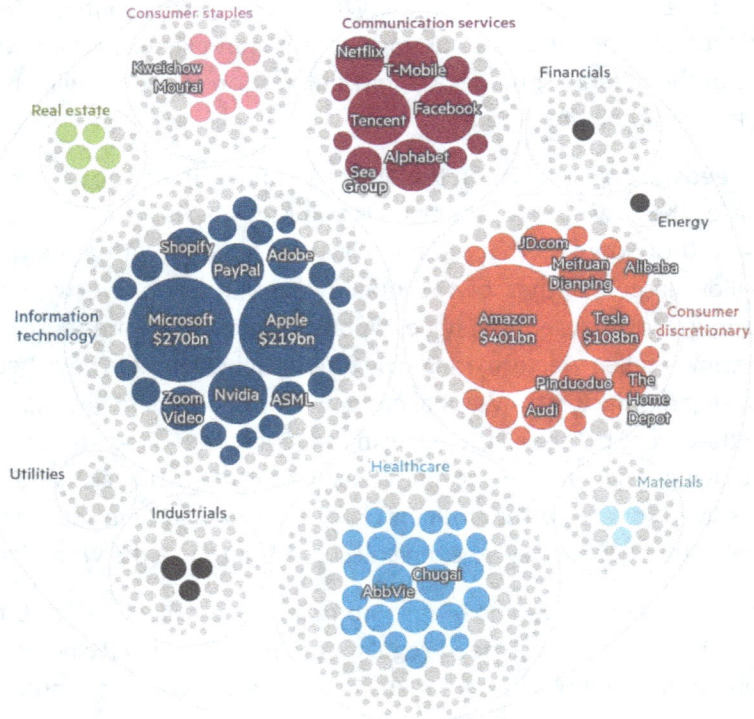

* As at Jun 17
Graphic: Alan Smith   Source: Capital IQ
© FT

# Appendix

## Covid-19 genome

```
   1 attaaaggtt tataccttcc caggtaacaa accaaccaac tttcgatctc ttgtagatct
  61 gttctctaaa cgaactttaa aatctgtgtg gctgtcactc ggctgcatgc ttagtgcact
 121 cacgcagtat aattaataac taattactgt cgttgacagg acacgagtaa ctcgtctatc
 181 ttctgcaggc tgcttacggt ttcgtccgtg ttgcagccga tcatcagcac atctaggttt
 241 cgtccgggtg tgaccgaaag gtaagatgga gagccttgtc cctggtttca acgagaaaac
 301 acacgtccaa ctcagtttgc ctgttttaca ggttcgcgac gtgctcgtac gtggctttgg
 361 agactccgtg gaggaggtct tatcagaggc acgtcaacat cttaaagatg gcacttgtgg
 421 cttagtagaa gttgaaaaag gcgttttgcc tcaacttgaa cagccctatg tgttcatcaa
 481 acgttcggat gctcgaactg cacctcatgg tcatgttatg gttgagctgg tagcagaact
 541 cgaaggcatt cagtacggtc gtagtggtga gacacttggt gtccttgtcc ctcatgtggg
 601 cgaaatacca gtggcttacc gcaaggttct tcttcgtaag aacggtaata aaggagctgg
 661 tggccatagt tacggcgccg atctaaagtc atttgactta ggcgacgagc ttggcactga
 721 tccttatgaa gattttcaag aaaactggaa cactaaacat agcagtggtg ttacccgtga
 781 actcatgcgt gagcttaacg agggggcata cactcgctat gtcgataaca acttctgtgg
 841 ccctgatggc taccctcttg agtgcattaa agaccttcta gcacgtgctg gtaaagcttc
 901 atgcactttg tccgaacaac tggactttat tgacactaag aggggtgtat actgctgccg
 961 tgaacatgag catgaaattg cttggtacac ggaacgttct gaaaagagct atgaattgca
1021 gacaccttt gaaattaaat tggcaaagaa atttgacacc ttcaatgggg aatgtccaaa
1081 ttttgtattt cccttaaatt ccataatcaa gactattcaa ccaaggggttg aaaagaaaaa
1141 gcttgatggc tttatgggta gaattcgatc tgtctatcca gttgcgtcac caaatgaatg
1201 caaccaaatg tgcctttcaa ctctcatgaa gtgtgatcat tgtggtgaaa cttcatggca
1261 gacgggcgat tttgttaaag ccacttgcga atttgtggc actgagaatt tgactaaaga
1321 aggtgccact acttgtggtt acttccccca aaatgctgtt gttaaatttt attgtccagc
1381 atgtcacaat tcagaagtag gacctgagca tagtcttgcc gaataccata tgaatctgg
1441 cttgaaaacc attcttcgta agggtggtcg cactattgcc tttggaggct gtgtgttctc
1501 ttatgttggt tgccataaca agtgtgccta ttgggttcca cgtgctagcg ctaacatagg
1561 ttgtaaccat acaggtgttg ttggagaagg ttccgaaggt cttaatgaca accttcttga
1621 aatactccaa aaagagaaag tcaacatcaa tattgttggt gactttaaac ttaatgaaga
1681 gatcgccatt atttggcat cttttctgc ttccacaagt gcttttgtgg aaactgtgaa
1741 aggtttggat tataaagcat caaacaaat tgttgaatcc tgtggtaatt ttaaagttac
1801 aaaaggaaaa gctaaaaaag gtgcctggaa tattggtgaa cagaaatcaa tactgagtcc
1861 tctttatgca tttgcatcag aggctgctcg tgttgtacga tcaattttct cccgcactct
1921 tgaaactgct caaaattctg tgcgtgtttt acagaaggcc gctataacaa tactagatgg
1981 aatttcacag tattcactga gactcattga tgctatgatg ttcacatctg atttggctac
2041 taacaatcta gttgtaatgg cctacattac aggtggtgtt gttcagttga cttcgcagtg
2101 gctaactaac atctttggca ctgtttatga aaaactcaaa cccgtccttg attggcttga
2161 agagaagttt aaggaaggtg tagagtttct tagagacggt tgggaaattg ttaaatttat
2221 ctcaacctgt gcttgtgaaa ttgtcggtgg acaaattgtc acctgtgcaa aggaaattaa
2281 ggagagtgtt cagacattct ttaagcttgt aaataaattt ttggctttgt gtgctgactc
2341 tatcattatt ggtggagcta aacttaaagc cttgaattta ggtgaaacat tgtcacgca
2401 ctcaaaggga ttgtacagaa agtgtgttaa atccagagaa gaaactggcc tactcatgcc
2461 tctaaaagcc ccaaaagaaa ttatcttctt agagggagaa acacttccca cagaagtgtt
2521 aacagaggaa gttgtcttga aaactggtga tttacaacca ttagaacaac ctactagtga
2581 agctgttgaa gctccattgg ttggtacacc agtttgtatt aacgggctta tgttgctcga
2641 aatcaaagac acagaaaagt actgtgccct tgcacctaat atgatggtaa caaacaatac
2701 cttcacactc aaaggcggtg caccaacaaa ggttactttt ggtgatgaca ctgtgataga
2761 agtgcaaggt tacaagagtg tgaatatcac ttttgaactt gatgaaagga ttgataaagt
2821 acttaatgag aagtgctctg cctatacagt tgaactcggt acagaagtaa atgagttcgc
2881 ctgtgttgtg gcagatgctg tcataaaaac tttgcaacca gtatctgaat tacttacacc
2941 actgggcatt gatttagatg agtggagtat ggctacatac tacttatttg atgagtctgg
3001 tgagtttaaa ttggcttcac atatgtattg ttctttctac cctccagatg aggatgaaga
3061 agaaggtgat tgtgaagaag aagagtttga gccatcaact caatatgagt atggtactga
3121 agatgattac caaggtaaac ctttggaatt tggtgccact tctgctgctc ttcaacctga
3181 agaagagcaa gaagaagatt ggttagatga tgatagtcaa caaactgttg gtcaacaaga
3241 cggcagtgag gacaatcaga caactactat tcaaacaatt gttgaggttc aacctcaatt
3301 agagatggaa cttacaccag ttgttcagac tattgaagtg aatagtttta gtggttattt
3361 aaaacttact gacaatgtat acattaaaaa tgcagacatt gtggaagaag ctaaaaaggt
3421 aaaaccaaca gtggttgtta atgcagccaa tgtttacctt aaacatggag gaggtgttgc
```

82

```
3481 aggagcctta aataaggcta ctaacaatgc catgcaagtt gaatctgatg attacatagc
3541 tactaatgga ccacttaaag tgggtggtag ttgtgtttta agcggacaca atcttgctaa
3601 acactgtctt catgttgtcg gcccaaatgt taacaaaggt gaagacattc aacttcttaa
3661 gagtgcttat gaaaatttta atcagcacga agttctactt gcaccattat tatcagctgg
3721 tattttggt gctgaccta tacattcttt aagagtttgt gtagatactg ttcgcacaaa
3781 tgtctactta gctgtctttg ataaaaatct ctatgacaaa cttgtttcaa gcttttgga
3841 aatgaagagt gaaaagcaag ttgaacaaaa gatcgctgag attcctaaag aggaagttaa
3901 gccatttata actgaaagta aaccttcagt tgaacagaga aaacaagatg ataagaaaat
3961 caaagcttgt gttgaagaag ttacaacaac tctggaagaa actaagttcc tcacagaaaa
4021 cttgttactt tatattgaca ttaatggcaa tcttcatcca gattctgcca ctcttgttag
4081 tgacattgac atcactttct aaagaaaga tgctccatat atagtgggtg atgttgttca
4141 agagggtgtt ttaactgctg tggttatacc tactaaaaag gctggtggca ctactgaaat
4201 gctagcgaaa gctttgagaa aagtgccaac agacaattat ataaccactt acccgggtca
4261 gggtttaaat ggttacactg tagaggaggc aaagacagtg cttaaaagt gtaaagtgc
4321 cttttacatt ctaccatcta ttatctctaa tgagaagcaa gaaattcttg gaactgtttc
4381 ttggaatttg cgagaaatgc ttgcacatgc agaagaaaca cgcaaattaa tgcctgtctg
4441 tgtggaaact aaagccatag tttcaactat acagcgtaaa tataagggta ttaaaataca
4501 agagggtgtg gttgattatg gtgctagatt ttactttac accagtaaaa caactgtagc
4561 gtcacttatc aacacactta acgatctaaa tgaaactctt gttacaatgc cacttggcta
4621 tgtaacacat ggcttaaatt tggaagaagc tgctcggtat atgagatctc tcaaagtgcc
4681 agctacagtt tctgtttctt cacctgatgc tgttacagcg tataatggtt atcttacttc
4741 ttcttctaaa acacctgaag aacattttat tgaaaccatc tcacttgctg gttcctataa
4801 agattggtcc tattctggac aatctacaca actaggtata gaatttctta agagaggtga
4861 taaagtgta tattcacta gtaatcctac cacattccac ctagatggtg aagttatcac
4921 ctttgacaat cttaagacac ttctttcttt gagagaagtg aggactatta aggtgtttac
4981 aacagtagac aacattaacc tccacacgca agttgtggac atgtcaatga catatggaca
5041 acagtttggt ccaacttatt tggatggagc tgatgttact aaaataaaac ctcataattc
5101 acatgaaggt aaaacatttt atgttttacc taatgatgac actctacgtg ttgaggcttt
5161 tgagtactac cacacaactg atcctagttt tctgggtagg tacatgtcag cattaaatca
5221 cactaaaaag tggaaatacc cacaagttaa tggtttaact tctattaaat gggcagataa
5281 caactgttat cttgccactg cattgttaac actccaacaa atagagttga agtttaatcc
5341 acctgctcta caagatgctt attacagagc aagggctggt gaagctgcta acttttgtgc
5401 acttatctta gcctactgta ataagacagt aggtgagtta ggtgatgtta gagaaacaat
5461 gagttacttg tttcaacatg ccaatttaga ttcttgcaaa agagtcttga acgtggtgtg
5521 taaaacttgt ggacaacagc agacaaccct taagggtgta gaagctgtta tgtacatggg
5581 cacactttct tatgaacaat ttaagaaagg tgttcagata ccttgtacgt gtggtaaaca
5641 agctacaaaa tatctagtac aacaggagtc accttttgtt atgatgtcag caccacctgc
5701 tcagtatgaa cttaagcatg gtacatttac ttgtgctagt gagtacactg gtaattacca
5761 gtgtggtcac tataaacata taacttctaa agaaactttg tattgcatag acggtgcttt
5821 acttacaaag tcctcagaat acaaaggtcc tattacggat gttttctaca aagaaaacag
5881 ttacacaaca accataaaac cagttactta taaattggat ggtgttgttt gtacagaaat
5941 tgaccctaag ttggacaatt attataagaa agacaattct tatttcacag agcaaccaat
6001 tgatcttgta ccaaaccaac catatccaaa cgcaagcttc gataatttta gtttgtatg
6061 tgataatatc aaatttgctg atgatttaaa ccagttaact ggttataaga aacctgcttc
6121 aagagagctt aaagttacat ttttccctga cttaaatggt gatgtggtgg ctattgatta
6181 taaacactac acaccctctt ttaagaaagg agctaaattg ttacataaac ctattgtttg
6241 gcatgttaac aatgcaacta ataaagccac gtataaacca aatacctggt gtatacgttg
6301 tctttggagc acaaaccag ttgaaacatc aaattcgttt gatgtactga agtcagagga
6361 cgcgcaggga atggataatc ttgcctgcga agatctaaaa ccagtctctg aagaagtagt
6421 ggaaaatcct accatacaga aagacgttct tgagtgtaat gtgaaaacta ccgaagttgt
6481 aggagacatt tacttaaaac cagcaaataa tagtttaaaa attacagaag aggttggcca
6541 cacagatcta atggctgctt atgtagacaa ttctagtctt actattaaga aacctaatga
6601 attatctaga gtattaggtt tgaaaaccct tgctactcat ggtttagctg ctgttaatag
6661 tgtcccttgg gatactatag ctaattatgc taagccttttt cttaacaaag ttgttagtac
6721 aactactaac atagttacac ggtgtttaaa ccgtgtttgt actaattata tgccttattt
6781 ctttactta ttgctacaat tgtgtacttt tactagaagt acaaattcta gaattaaagc
6841 atctatgccg actactatag caaagaatac tgttaagagt gtcggtaaat tttgtctaga
6901 ggcttcatt aattatttga agtcacctaa ttttctaaaa ctgataaata ttataatttg
6961 gttttacta ttaagtgttt gcctaggttc tttaatctac tcaaccgctg ctttaggtgt
7021 tttaatgtct aatttaggca tgccttctta ctgtactggt tacagagaag ctatttgaa
7081 ctctactaat gtcactattg caacctactg tactggttct ataccttgta gtgtttgtct
```

83

```
 7141 tagtggttta gattctttag acacctatcc ttctttagaa actatacaaa ttaccatttc
 7201 atctttaaaa tgggatttaa ctgcttttgg cttagttgca gagtggtttt tggcatatat
 7261 tcttttcact aggttttct atgtacttgg attggctgca atcatgcaat tgtttttcag
 7321 ctattttgca gtacatttta ttagtaattc ttggcttatg tggttaataa ttaatcttgt
 7381 acaaatggcc ccgatttcag ctatggttag aatgtacatc ttctttgcat cattttatta
 7441 tgtatggaaa agttatgtgc atgttgtaga cggttgtaat tcatcaactt gtatgatgtg
 7501 ttacaaacgt aatagagcaa caagagtcga atgtacaact attgttaatg gtgttagaag
 7561 gtcctttat gtctatgcta atggaggtaa aggcttttgc aaactacaca attggaattg
 7621 tgttaattgt gatacattct gtgctggtag tacatttatt agtgatgaag ttgcgagaga
 7681 cttgtcacta cagtttaaaa gaccaataaa tcctactgac cagtcttctt acatcgttga
 7741 tagtgttaca gtgaagaatg gttccatcca tctttacttt gataaagctg gtcaaaagac
 7801 ttatgaaaga cattctctct ctcattttgt taacttagac aacctgagag ctaataacac
 7861 taaaggttca ttgcctatta atgttatagt ttttgatggt aaatcaaaat gtgaagaatc
 7921 atctgcaaaa tcagcgtctg tttactacag tcagcttatg tgtcaaccta tactgttact
 7981 agatcaggca ttagtgtctg atgttggtga tagtgcggaa gttgcagtta aatgtttga
 8041 tgcttacgtt aatacgtttt catcaacttt taacgtacca atggaaaaac tcaaaacact
 8101 agttgcaact gcagaagctg aacttgcaaa gaatgtgtcc ttagacaatg tcttatctac
 8161 ttttatttca gcagctcggc aagggtttgt tgattcagat gtagaaacta agatgttgt
 8221 tgaatgtctt aaattgtcac atcaatctga catagaagtt actggcgata gttgtaataa
 8281 ctatatgctc acctataaca aagttgaaaa catgacaccc cgtgaccttg gtgcttgtat
 8341 tgactgtagt gcgcgtcata ttaatgcgca ggtagcaaaa agtcacaaca ttgctttgat
 8401 atggaacgtt aaagatttca tgtcattgtc tgaacaacta cgaaaacaaa tacgtagtgc
 8461 tgctaaaaag aataacttac cttttaagtt gacatgtgca actactagac aagttgttaa
 8521 tgttgtaaca acaaagatag cacttaaggg tggtaaaatt gttaataatt ggttgaagca
 8581 gttaattaaa gttacacttg tgttcctttt tgttgctgct attttctatt taataacacc
 8641 tgttcatgtc atgtctaaac atactgactt ttcaagtgaa atcataggat acaaggctat
 8701 tgatggtggt gtcactcgtg acatagcatc tacagatact tgttttgcta caaacatgc
 8761 tgattttgac acatggttta gccagcgtgg tggtagttat actaatgaca aagcttgccc
 8821 attgattgct gcagtcataa caagagaagt gggttttgtc gtgcctggtt tgcctggcac
 8881 gatattacgc acaactaatg gtgacttttt gcatttctta cctagagttt ttagtgcagt
 8941 tggtaacatc tgttacacac catcaaaact tatagagtac actgactttg caacatcagc
 9001 ttgtgttttg gctgctgaat gtacaatttt taaagatgct tctggtaagc cagtaccata
 9061 ttgttatgat accaatgtac tagaaggttc tgttgcttat gaaagtttac gccctgacac
 9121 acgttatgtg ctcatggatg gctctattat tcaatttcct aacacctacc ttgaaggttc
 9181 tgttagagtg gtaacaactt ttgattctga gtactgtagg cacggcactt gtgaaagatc
 9241 agaagctggt gtttgtgtat ctactagtgg tagatgggta cttaacaatg attattacag
 9301 atctttacca ggagttttct gtggtgtaga tgctgtaaat ttacttacta atatgtttac
 9361 accactaatt caacctattg gtgctttgga catatcagca tctatagtag ctggtggtat
 9421 tgtagctatc gtagtaacat gccttgccta ctatttatg aggtttagaa gagcttttgg
 9481 tgaatacagt catgtagttg cctttaatac tttactattc cttatgtcat tcactgtact
 9541 ctgtttaaca ccagtttact cattcttacc tggtgtttat tctgttatttt acttgtactt
 9601 gacattttat cttactaatg atgtttcttt tttagcacat attcagtgga tggttatgtt
 9661 cacacctta gtacctttct ggataacaat tgcttatatc atttgtattt ccacaaagca
 9721 tttctattgg ttctttagta attacctaaa gagacgtgta gtctttaatg gtgtttcctt
 9781 tagtactttt gaagaagctg cgctgtgcac ctttttgtta aataaagaaa tgtatctaaa
 9841 gttgcgtagt gatgtgctat tacctcttac gcaatataat agatacttag ctctttataa
 9901 taagtacaag tattttagtg gagcaatgga tacaactagc tacagagaag ctgcttgttg
 9961 tcatctcgca aaggctctca atgacttcag taactcaggt tctgatgttc tttaccaacc
10021 accacaaacc tctatcacct cagctgtttt gcagagtggt tttagaaaaa tggcattccc
10081 atctggtaaa gttgagggtt gtatggtaca agtaacttgt ggtacaacta cacttaacgg
10141 tctttggctt gatgacgtag tttactgtcc aagacatgtg atctgcacct ctgaagacat
10201 gcttaaccct aattatgaag atttactcat tcgtaagtct aatcataatt cttggtaca
10261 ggctggtaat gttcaactca gggttattgg acattctatg caaattgtg tacttaagct
10321 taaggttgat acagccaatc ctaagacacc taagtataag tttgttcgca ttcaaccagg
10381 acagactttt tcagtgttag cttgttacaa tggttcacca tctggtgttt accaatgtgc
10441 tatgaggccc aatttcacta ttaagggttc attccttaat ggttcatgtg gtagtgttgg
10501 ttttaacata gattatgact gtgtctcttt tgttacatg caccatatgg aattaccaac
10561 tggagttcat gctggcacag acttagaagg taacttttat ggacctttg ttgacaggca
10621 aacagcacaa gcagctggta cggacacaac tattacagtt aatgttttag cttggttgta
10681 cgctgctgtt ataaatggag acaggtggtt tctcaatcga tttaccacaa ctcttaatga
10741 ctttaacctt gtggctatga agtacaatta tgaacctcta acacaagacc atgttgacat
```

```
10801 actaggacct ctttctgctc aaactggaat tgccgtttta gatatgtgtg cttcattaaa
10861 agaattactg caaaatggta tgaatggacg taccatattg ggtagtgctt tattagaaga
10921 tgaatttaca ccttttgatg ttgttagaca atgctcaggt gttactttcc aaagtgcagt
10981 gaaaagaaca atcaagggta cacaccactg gttgttactc acaattttga cttcactttt
11041 agttttagtc cagagtactc aatggtcttt gttcttttt ttgtatgaaa atgccttttt
11101 accttttgct atgggtatta ttgctatgtc tgcttttgca atgatgtttg tcaaacataa
11161 gcatgcattt ctctgtttgt ttttgttacc ttctcttgcc actgtagctt attttaatat
11221 ggtctatatg cctgctagtt gggtgatgcg tattatgaca tggttggata tggttgatac
11281 tagtttgtct ggttttaagc taaaagactg tgttatgtat gcatcagctg tagtgttact
11341 aatccttatg acagcaagaa ctgtgtatga tgatggtgct aggagagtgt ggacacttat
11401 gaatgtcttg acactcgttt ataaagttta ttatggtaat gctttagatc aagccatttc
11461 catgtgggct cttataatct ctgttacttc taactactca ggtgtagtta caactgtcat
11521 gttttggcc agaggtattg tttttatgtg tgttgagtat tgccctattt tcttcataac
11581 tggtaataca cttcagtgta taatgctagt ttattgtttc ttaggctatt tttgtacttg
11641 ttactttggc ctcttttgtt tactcaaccg ctactttaga ctgactcttg gtgtttatga
11701 ttacttagtt tctacacagg agtttagata tatgaattca caggactac tcccacccaa
11761 gaatagcata gatgccttca aactcaacat taaattgttg ggtgttggtg gcaaaccttg
11821 tatcaaagta gccactgtac agtctaaaat gtcagatgta aagtgcacat cagtagtctt
11881 actctcagtt ttgcaacaac tcagagtaga atcatcatct aaattgtggg ctcaatgtgt
11941 ccagttacac aatgacattc tcttagctaa agatactact gaagcctttg aaaaaatggt
12001 ttcactactt tctgttttgc tttccatgca gggtgctgta gacataaaca gctttgtga
12061 agaaatgctg gacaacaggg caaccttaca agctatagcc tcagagttta gttcccttcc
12121 atcatatgca gcttttgcta ctgctcaaga agcttatgag caggctgttg ctaatggtga
12181 ttctgaagtt gttcttaaaa agttgaagaa gtctttgaat gtggctaaat ctgaatttga
12241 ccgtgatgca gccatgcaac gtaagttgga aaagatggct gatcaagcta tgacccaaat
12301 gtataaacag gctagatctg aggacaagag ggcaaaagtt actagtgcta tgcagacaat
12361 gcttttcact atgcttagaa agttggataa tgatgcactc aacaacatta tcaacaatgc
12421 aagagatggt tgtgttccct tgaacataat acctcttaca acagcagcca aactaatggt
12481 tgtcatacca gactataaca catataaaaa tacgtgtgat ggtacaacat ttacttatgc
12541 atcagcattg tgggaaatcc aacaggttgt agatgcagat agtaaaattg ttcaacttag
12601 tgaaattagt atggacaatt cacctaattt agcatggcct cttattgtaa cagctttaag
12661 ggccaattct gctgtcaaat tacagaataa tgagcttagt cctgttgcac tacgacagat
12721 gtcttgtgct gccggtacta cacaaactgc ttgcactgat gacaatgcgt tagcttacta
12781 caacacaaca aagggaggta ggtttgtact tgcactgtta tccgatttac aggatttgaa
12841 atgggctaga ttccctaaga gtgatggaac tggtactatc tatacagaac tggaaccacc
12901 ttgtaggttt gttacagaca cacctaaagg tcctaaagtg aagtatttat actttattaa
12961 aggattaaac aacctaaata gaggtatggt acttggtagt ttagctgcca cagtacgtct
13021 acaagctggt aatgcaacag aagtgcctgc caattcaact gtattatctt tctgtgcttt
13081 tgctgtagat gctgctaaag cttacaaaga ttatctagct agtgggggac aaccaatcac
13141 taattgtgtt aagatgttgt gtacacacac tggtactggt caggcaataa cagttacacc
13201 ggaagccaat atggatcaag aatcctttgg tggtgcatcg tgttgtctgt actgccgttg
13261 ccacatagat catccaaatc ctaaaggatt ttgtgactta aaaggtaagt atgtacaaat
13321 acctacaact tgtgctaatg accctgtggg ttttacactt aaaaacacag tctgtaccgt
13381 ctgcggtatg tggaaaggtt atggctgtag ttgtgatcaa ctccgcgaac ccatgcttca
13441 gtcagctgat gcacaatcgt ttttaaacgg gtttgcggtg taagtgcagc ccgtcttaca
13501 ccgtgcggca caggcactag tactgatgtc gtatacaggg cttttgacat ctacaatgat
13561 aaagtagctg gttttgctaa attcctaaaa actaattgtt gtcgcttcca agaaaaggac
13621 gaagatgaca attaattga ttcttacttt gtagttaaga gacacacttt ctctaactac
13681 caacatgaag aaacaattta taatttactt aaggattgtc cagctgttgc taaacatgac
13741 ttctttaagt ttagaataga cggtgacatg gtaccacata tatcacgtca acgtcttact
13801 aaatacacaa tggcagacct cgtctatgct ttaaggcatt ttgatgaagg taattgtgac
13861 acattaaaag aaatacttgt cacatacaat tgttgtgatg atgattattt caataaaaag
13921 gactggtatg atttgtaga aaacccagat atattacgcg tatacgccaa cttaggtgaa
13981 cgtgtacgcc aagctttgtt aaaaacagta caattctgtg atgccatgcg aaatgctggt
14041 attgttggtg tactgacatt agataatcaa gatctcaatg gtaactggta tgatttcggt
14101 gatttcatac aaaccacgcc aggtagtgga gttcctgttg tagattctta ttattcattg
14161 ttaatgccta tattaacctt gaccagggct ttaactgcag agtcacatgt tgacactgac
14221 ttaacaaagc cttacattaa gtgggatttg ttaaaatatg acttcacgga agagaggtta
14281 aaactctttg accgttattt taaatattgg gatcagacat accacccaaa ttgtgttaac
14341 tgtttggatg acagatgcat tctgcattgt gcaaacttta atgtttatt ctctacagtg
14401 ttcccaccta caagttttgg accactagtg agaaaaatat ttgttgatgg tgttccattt
```

```
14461 gtagtttcaa ctggatacca cttcagagag ctaggtgttg tacataatca ggatgtaaac
14521 ttacatagct ctagacttag ttttaaggaa ttacttgtgt atgctgctga ccctgctatg
14581 cacgctgctt ctggtaatct attactagat aaacgcacta cgtgcttttc agtagctgca
14641 cttactaaca atgttgcttt tcaaactgtc aaacccggta atttttaacaa agacttctat
14701 gactttgctg tgtctaaggg tttctttaag gaaggaagtt ctgttgaatt aaaacacttc
14761 ttctttgctc aggatggtaa tgctgctatc agcgattatg actactatcg ttataatcta
14821 ccaacaatgt gtgatatcag acaactacta tttgtagttg aagttgttga taagtacttt
14881 gattgttacg atggtggctg tattaatgct aaccaagtca tcgtcaacaa cctagacaaa
14941 tcagctggtt ttccatttaa taaatggggt aaggctagac tttattatga ttcaatgagt
15001 tatgaggatc aagatgcact tttcgcatat acaaaacgta atgtcatccc tactataact
15061 caaatgaatc ttaagtatgc cattagtgca aagaatagag ctcgcaccgt agctggtgtc
15121 tctatctgta gtactatgac caatagacag tttcatcaaa aattattgaa atcaatagcc
15181 gccactagag gagctactgt agtaattgga acaagcaaat tctatggtgg ttggcacaac
15241 atgttaaaaa ctgtttatag tgatgtagaa aaccctcacc ttatggggtg ggattatcct
15301 aaatgtgata gagccatgcc taacatgctt agaattatgg cctcacttgt tcttgctcgc
15361 aaacatacaa cgtgttgtag cttgtcacac cgtttctata gattagctaa tgagtgtgct
15421 caagtattga gtgaaatggt catgtgtggc ggttcactat atgttaaacc aggtggaacc
15481 tcatcaggag atgccacaac tgcttatgct aatagtgttt ttaacatttg tcaagctgtc
15541 acggccaatg ttaatgcact tttatctact gatggtaaca aaattgccga taagtatgtc
15601 cgcaatttac aacacagact ttatgagtgt ctctatagaa atagagatgt tgacacagac
15661 tttgtgaatg agttttacgc atatttgcgt aaacatttct caatgatgat actctctgac
15721 gatgctgttg tgtgtttcaa tagcacttat gcatctcaag gtctagtggc tagcataaag
15781 aactttaagt cagttcttta ttatcaaaac aatgtttta tgtctgaagc aaaatgttgg
15841 actgagactg accttactaa aggacctcat gaattttgct ctcaacatac aatgctagtt
15901 aaacagggtg atgattatgt gtaccttcct tacccagatc catcaagaat cctaggggcc
15961 ggctgttttg tagatgatat cgtaaaaaca gatggtacac ttatgattga acggttcgtg
16021 tctttagcta tagatgctta cccacttact aaacatccta atcaggagta tgctgatgtc
16081 tttcatttgt acttacaata cataagaaag ctacatgatg agttaacagg acacatgtta
16141 gacatgtatt ctgttatgct tactaatgat aacacttcaa ggtattggga acctgagttt
16201 tatgaggcta tgtacacacc gcatacagtc ttacaggctg ttggggcttg tgttctttgc
16261 aattcacaga cttcattaag atgtggtgct tgcatacgta gaccattctt atgttgtaaa
16321 tgctgttacg accatgtcat atcaacatca cataaattag tcttgtctgt taatccgtat
16381 gtttgcaatg ctccaggttg tgatgtcaca gatgtgactc aactttactt aggaggtatg
16441 agctattatt gtaaatcaca taaaccaccc attagttttc cattgtgtgc taatggacaa
16501 gttttggtt tatataaaaa tacatgtgtt ggtagcgata atgttactga ctttaatgca
16561 attgcaacat gtgactggac aaatgctggt gattacattt tagctaacac ctgtactgaa
16621 agactcaagc ttttgcagc agaaacgctc aaagctactg aggagacatt taaactgtct
16681 tatggtattg ctactgtacg tgaagtgctg tctgacagag aattacatct ttcatgggaa
16741 gttggtaaac ctagaccacc acttaaccga aattatgtct ttactggtta tcgtgtaact
16801 aaaaacagta agtacaaat aggagagtac acctttgaaa aaggtgacta tggtgatgct
16861 gttgtttacc gaggtacaac aacttacaaa ttaaatgttg gtgattattt tgtgctgaca
16921 tcacatacag taatgccatt aagtgcacct acactagtgc cacaagagca ctatgttaga
16981 attactggct tatacccaac actcaatatc tcagatgagt tttctagcaa tgttgcaaat
17041 tatcaaaagg ttggtatgca aaagtattct acactccagg gaccacctgg tactggtaag
17101 agtcattttg ctattggcct agctctctac taccccttctg ctcgcatagt gtatacagct
17161 tgctctcatg ccgctgttga tgcactatgt gagaaggcat taaaatattt gcctatagat
17221 aaatgtagta gaattatacc tgcacgtgct cgtgtagagt gttttgataa attcaaagtg
17281 aattcaacat tagaacagta tgtcttttgt actgtaaatg cattgcctga cgacagca
17341 gatatagttg tctttgatga aatttcaatg gccacaaatt atgatttgag tgttgtcaat
17401 gccagattac gtgctaagca ctatgtgtac attggcgacc ctgctcaatt acctgcacca
17461 cgcacattgc taactaaggg cacactagaa ccagaatatt tcaattcagt gtgtagactt
17521 atgaaaacta taggtccaga catgttcctc ggaacttgtc ggcgttgtcc tgctgaaatt
17581 gttgacactg tgagtgcttt ggtttatgat aataagctta agcacataa agacaaatca
17641 gctcaatgct ttaaaatgtt ttataagggt gttatcacgc atgatgtttc atctgcaatt
17701 aacaggccac aaataggcgt ggtaagagaa ttccttacac gtaaccctgc ttggagaaaa
17761 gctgtcttta tttcaccttta taattcacag aatgctgtag cctcaaagat tttgggacta
17821 ccaactcaaa ctgttgattc atcacaggc tcagaatatg actatgtcat attcactcaa
17881 accactgaaa cagctcactc ttgtaatgta aacagattta atgttgctat taccagagca
17941 aaagtaggca tactttgcat aatgtctgat agagaccttt atgacaagtt gcaatttaca
18001 agtcttgaaa ttccacgtag gaatgtggca actttacaag ctgaaaatgt aacaggactc
18061 tttaaagatt gtagtaaggt aatcactggg ttacatccta cacaggcacc tacacacctc
```

```
18121 agtgttgaca ctaaattcaa aactgaaggt ttatgtgttg acatacctgg catacctaag
18181 gacatgacct atagaagact catctctatg atgggtttta aaatgaatta tcaagttaat
18241 ggttacccta acatgtttat cacccgcgaa gaagctataa gacatgtacg tgcatggatt
18301 ggcttcgatg tcgagggtg tcatgctact agagaagctg ttggtaccaa tttaccttta
18361 cagctaggtt tttctacagg tgttaaccta gttgctgtac ctacaggtta tgttgataca
18421 cctaataata cagattttc cagagttagt gctaaaccac cgcctggaga tcaatttaaa
18481 cacctcatac cacttatgta caaaggactt ccttggaatg tagtgcgtat aaagattgta
18541 caaatgttaa gtgacacact taaaaatctc tctgacagag tcgtatttgt cttatgggca
18601 catggctttg agttgacatc tatgaagtat tttgtgaaaa taggacctga gcgcacctgt
18661 tgtctatgtg atagacgtgc cacatgcttt tccactgctt cagacactta tgcctgttgg
18721 catcattcta ttggatttga ttacgtctat aatccgttta tgattgatgt caacaatgg
18781 ggttttacag gtaacctaca aagcaaccat gatctgtatt gtcaagtcca tggtaatgca
18841 catgtagcta gttgtgatgc aatcatgact aggtgtctag ctgtccacga gtgctttgtt
18901 aagcgtgttg actggactat tgaatatcct ataattggtg atgaactgaa gattaatgcg
18961 gcttgtagaa aggttcaaca catggttgtt aaagctgcat tattagcaga caaattccca
19021 gttcttcacg acattggtaa ccctaaagct attaagtgtg tacctcaagc tgatgtagaa
19081 tggaagttct atgatgcaca gccttgtagt gacaaagctt ataaaataga agaattattc
19141 tattcttatg ccacacattc tgacaaattc acagatggtg tatgcctatt ttggaattgc
19201 aatgtcgata gatatcctgc taattccatt gtttgtagat ttgacactag agtgctatct
19261 aaccttaact tgcctggttg tgatggtggc agtttgtatg taaataaaca tgcattccac
19321 acaccagctt ttgataaaag tgcttttgtt aatttaaaac aattaccatt tttctattac
19381 tctgacagtc catgtgagtc tcatggaaaa caagtagtgt cagatataga ttatgtacca
19441 ctaaagtctg ctacgtgtat aacacgttgc aatttaggtg gtgctgtctg tagacatcat
19501 gctaatgagt acagattgta tctcgatgct tataacatga tgatctcagc tggctttagc
19561 ttgtgggttt acaaacaatt tgatacttat aacctctgga acacttttac aagacttcag
19621 agtttagaaa atgtggcttt taatgttgta aataagggac actttgatgg acaacagggt
19681 gaagtaccag tttctatcat taataacact gtttacacaa aagttgatgg tgttgatgta
19741 gaattgtttg aaaataaaac aacattacct gttaatgtag catttgagct ttgggctaag
19801 cgcaacatta accagtacc agaggtgaaa atactcaata atttgggtgt ggacattgct
19861 gctaatactg tgatctggga ctacaaaaga gatgctccag cacatatatc tactattggt
19921 gtttgttcta tgactgacat agccaagaaa ccaactgaaa cgatttgtgc accactcact
19981 gtcttttttg atggtagagt tgatggtcaa gtagacttat ttagaaatgc ccgtaatggt
20041 gttcttatta cagaaggtag tgttaaaggt ttacaaccat ctgtaggtcc caaacaagct
20101 agtcttaatg gagtcacatt aattggagaa gccgtaaaaa cacagttcaa ttattataag
20161 aaagttgatg gtgttgtcca acaattacct gaaacttact ttactcagag tagaaattta
20221 caagaattta acccaggag tcaaatggaa attgatttct tagaattagc tatggatgaa
20281 ttcattgaac ggtataaatt agaaggctat gccttcgaac atatcgttta tggagatttt
20341 agtcatagtc agttaggtgg tttacatcta ctgattggac tagctaaacg ttttaaggaa
20401 tcaccttttg aattagaaga ttttattcct atggacagta cagttaaaaa ctatttcata
20461 acagatgcgc aaacaggttc atctaagtgt gtgtgttctg ttattgattt attacttgat
20521 gattttgttg aaataataaa atcccaagat ttatctgtag tttctaaggt tgtcaaagtg
20581 actattgact atacagaaat ttcatttatg ctttggtgta aagatggcca tgtagaaaca
20641 ttttacccaa aattacaatc tagtcaagcg tggcaaccgg gtgttgctat gcctaatctt
20701 tacaaaatgc aagaatgct attagaaaag tgtgaccttc aaaattatgg tgatagtgca
20761 acattaccta aaggcataat gatgaatgtc gcaaaatata ctcaactgtg tcaatattta
20821 aacacattaa cattagctgt accctataat atgagagtta tacattttgg tgctggttct
20881 gataaaggag ttgcaccagg tacagctgtt ttaagacagt ggttgcctac gggtacgctg
20941 cttgtcgatt cagatcttaa tgactttgtc tctgatgcag attcaacttt gattggtgat
21001 tgtgcaactg tacatacagc taataaatgg gatctcatta ttagtgatat gtacgaccct
21061 aagactaaaa atgttacaaa agaaaatgac tctaaagagg gttttttcac ttacatttgt
21121 gggtttatac aacaaagct agctcttgga ggttccgtgg ctataaagat aacagaacat
21181 tcttggaatg ctgatctta taagctcatg ggacacttcg catggtggac agcctttgtt
21241 actaatgtga atgcgtcatc atctgaagca tttttaattg gatgtaatta tcttggcaaa
21301 ccacgcgaac aaatagatgg ttatgtcatg catgcaaatt acatattttg gaggaataca
21361 aatccaattc agttgtcttc ctattcttta tttgacatga gtaaatttcc ccttaaatta
21421 aggggtactg ctgttatgtc tttaaaagaa ggtcaaatca atgatatgat tttatctctt
21481 cttagtaaag gtagacttat aattagagaa aacaacagag ttgttatttc tagtgatgtt
21541 cttgttaaca actaaacgaa caatgtttgt ttttcttgtt ttattgccac tagtctctag
21601 tcagtgtgtt aatcttacaa ccagaactca attaccccct gcatacacta attctttcac
21661 acgtggtgtt tattaccctg acaaagtttt cagatcctca gttttacatt caactcagga
21721 cttgttctta cctttctttt ccaatgttac ttggttccat gctatacatg tctctgggac
```

```
21781 caatggtact aagaggtttg ataaccctgt cctaccattt aatgatggtg tttattttgc
21841 ttccactgag aagtctaaca taataagagg ctggatttttt ggtactactt tagattcgaa
21901 gacccagtcc ctacttattg ttaataacgc tactaatgtt gttattaaag tctgtgaatt
21961 tcaattttgt aatgatccat ttttgggtgt ttattaccac aaaaacaaca aaagttggat
22021 ggaaagtgag ttcagagttt attctagtgc gaataattgc acttttgaat atgtctctca
22081 gccttttctt atggaccttg aaggaaaaca gggtaatttc aaaaatctta ggaatttgt
22141 gtttaagaat attgatggtt attttaaaat atattctaag cacacgccta ttaatttagt
22201 gcgtgatctc cctcagggtt tttcggcttt agaaccattg gtagatttgc caataggtat
22261 taacatcact aggtttcaaa ctttacttgc tttacataga agttatttga ctcctggtga
22321 ttcttcttca ggttggacag ctggtgctgc agcttattat gtgggttatc ttcaacctag
22381 gacttttcta ttaaaatata atgaaaatgg aaccattaca gatgctgtag actgtgcact
22441 tgaccctctc tcagaaacaa agtgtacgtt gaaatccttc actgtagaaa aaggaatcta
22501 tcaaacttct aactttagag tccaaccaac agaatctatt gttagatttc ctaatattac
22561 aaacttgtgc ccttttggtg aagtttttaa cgccaccaga tttgcatctg tttatgcttg
22621 gaacaggaag agaatcagca actgtgttgc tgattattct gtcctatata attccgcatc
22681 attttccact tttaagtgtt atggagtgtc tcctactaaa ttaaatgatc tctgctttac
22741 taatgtctat gcagattcat ttgtaattag aggtgatgaa gtcagacaaa tcgctccagg
22801 gcaaactgga aagattgctg attataatta taaattacca gatgattta caggctgcgt
22861 tatagcttgg aattctaaca atcttgattc taaggttggt ggtaattata attacctgta
22921 tagattgttt aggaagtcta atctcaaacc ttttgagaga gatatttcaa ctgaaatcta
22981 tcaggccggt agcacacctt gtaatggtgt tgaaggtttt aattgttact ttccctttaca
23041 atcatatggt ttccaaccca ctaatggtgt tggttaccaa ccatacagag tagtagtact
23101 ttcttttgaa cttctacatg caccagcaac tgtttgtgga cctaaaaagt ctactaatt
23161 ggttaaaaac aaatgtgtca atttcaactt caatggttta acaggcacag gtgttcttac
23221 tgagtctaac aaaaagtttc tgcctttcca acaatttggc agagacattg ctgacactac
23281 tgatgctgtc cgtgatccac agacacttga gattcttgac attacaccat gttcttttgg
23341 tggtgtcagt gttataacac caggaacaaa tacttctaac caggttgctg ttctttatca
23401 ggatgttaac tgcacagaag tccctgttgc tattcatgca gatcaactta ctcctacttg
23461 gcgtgtttat tctacaggtt ctaatgtttt tcaaacacgt gcaggctgtt taatagggc
23521 tgaacatgtc aacaactcat atgagtgtga catacccatt ggtgcaggta tatgcgctag
23581 ttatcagact cagactaatt ctcctcggcg ggcacgtagt gtagctagtc aatccatcat
23641 tgcctacact atgtcacttg gtgcagaaaa ttcagttgct tactctaata actctattgc
23701 catacccaca aattttacta ttagtgttac cacagaaatt ctaccagtgt ctatgaccaa
23761 gacatcagta gattgtacaa tgtacatttg tggtgattca actgaatgca gcaatctttt
23821 gttgcaatat ggcagttttt gtacacaatt aaaccgtgct ttaactggaa tagctgttga
23881 acaagacaaa aacacccaag aagttttgc acaagtcaaa caaatttaca aaacaccacc
23941 aattaaagat tttggtggtt ttaattttc acaaatatta ccagatccat caaaaccaag
24001 caagaggtca tttattgaag atctactttt caacaaagtg acacttgcag atgctggctt
24061 catcaaacaa tatggtgatt gccttggtga tattgctgct agagacctca tttgtgcaca
24121 aaagtttaac ggccttactg ttttgccacc tttgctcaca gatgaaatga ttgctcaata
24181 cacttctgca ctgttagcgg gtacaatcac ttctggttgg acctttggtg caggtgctgc
24241 attacaaata ccatttgcta tgcaaatggc ttataggttt aatggtattg gagttacaca
24301 gaatgttctc tatgagaacc aaaaaattgat tgccaaccaa tttaatagtg ctattggcaa
24361 aattcaagac tcactttctt ccacagcaag tgcacttgga aaacttcaag atgtggtcaa
24421 ccaaaatgca caagctttaa acacgcttgt taaacaactt agctccaatt ttggtgcaat
24481 ttcaagtgtt ttaaatgata tccttttcacg tcttgacaaa gttgaggctg aagtgcaaat
24541 tgataggttg atcacaggca gacttcaaag tttgcagaca tatgtgactc aacaattaat
24601 tagagctgca gaaatcagag cttctgctaa tcttgctgct actaaaatgt cagagtgtgt
24661 acttggacaa tcaaaaagag ttgatttttg tggaaagggc tatcatctta tgtccttccc
24721 tcagtcagca cctcatggtg tagtcttctt gcatgtgact tatgtccctg cacaagaaaa
24781 gaacttcaca actgctcctg ccatttgtca tgatggaaaa gcacacttc ctcgtgaagg
24841 tgtctttgtt tcaaatggca cacactggtt tgtaacacaa aggaattttt atgaaccaca
24901 aatcattact acagacaaca catttgtgtc tggtaactgt gatgttgtaa taggaattgt
24961 caacaacaca gtttatgatc ctttgcaacc tgaattagac tcattcaagg aggagttaga
25021 taaatatttt aagaatcata catcaccaga tgttgattta ggtgacatct ctggcattaa
25081 tgcttcagtt gtaaacattc aaaaagaaat tgaccgcctc aatgaggttg ccaagaattt
25141 aaatgaatct ctcatcgatc tccaagaact ggaaagtat gagcagtata taaaatggcc
25201 atggtacatt tggctaggtt ttatagctgg cttgattgcc atagtaatgg tgacaattat
25261 gctttgctgt atgaccagtt gctgtagttg tctcaagggc tgttgttctt gtggatcctg
25321 ctgcaaattt gatgaagacg actctgagcc agtgctcaaa ggagtcaaat tacattacac
25381 ataaacgaac ttatggattt gtttatgaga atcttcacaa ttggaactgt aactttgaag
```

```
25441 caaggtgaaa tcaaggatgc tactccttca gattttgttc gcgctactgc aacgataccg
25501 atacaagcct cactcccttt cggatggctt attgttggcg ttgcacttct tgctgttttt
25561 cagagcgctt ccaaaatcat aaccctcaaa aagagatggc aactagcact ctccaagggt
25621 gttcactttg tttgcaactt gctgttgttg tttgtaacag tttactcaca ccttttgctc
25681 gttgctgctg gccttgaagc ccctttttctc tatctttatg ctttagtcta cttcttgcag
25741 agtataaact ttgtaagaat aataatgagg ctttggcttt gctggaaatg ccgttccaaa
25801 aacccattac tttatgatgc caactatttt ctttgctggc atactaattg ttacgactat
25861 tgtatacctt acaatagtgt aacttcttca attgtcatta cttcaggtga tggcacaaca
25921 agtcctattt ctgaacatga ctaccagatt ggtggttata ctgaaaaatg ggaatctgga
25981 gtaaaagact gtgttgtatt acacagttac ttcacttcag actattacca gctgtactca
26041 actcaattga gtacagacac tggtgttgaa catgttacct tcttcatcta caataaaatt
26101 gttgatgagc ctgaagaaca tgtccaaatt cacacaatcg acggttcatc cggagttgtt
26161 aatccagtaa tggaaccaat ttatgatgaa ccgacgacga ctactagcgt gcctttgtaa
26221 gcacaagctg atgagtacga acttatgtac tcattcgttt cggaagagac aggtacgtta
26281 atagttaata gcgtacttct ttttcttgct ttcgtggtat tcttgctagt tacactagcc
26341 atccttactg cgcttcgatt gtgtgcgtac tgctgcaata ttgttaacgt gagtcttgta
26401 aaaccttctt tttacgttta ctctcgtgtt aaaaatctga attcttctag agttcctgat
26461 cttctggtct aaacgaacta aatattatat tagttttttct gtttggaact ttaattttag
26521 ccatggcaga ttccaacggt actattaccg ttgaagagct taaaaagctc cttgaacaat
26581 ggaacctagt aataggtttc ctattcctta catggatttg tcttctacaa tttgcctatg
26641 ccaacaggaa taggttttttg tatataatta agttaatttt cctctggctg ttatggccag
26701 taactttagc ttgttttgtg cttgctgctg tttacagaat aaattggatc accggtggaa
26761 ttgctatcgc aatggcttgt cttgtaggct tgatgtggct cagctacttc attgcttctt
26821 tcagactgtt tgcgcgtacg cgttccatgt ggtcattcaa tccagaaact aacattcttc
26881 tcaacgtgcc actccatggc actattctga ccagaccgct tctagaaagt gaactcgtaa
26941 tcggagctgt gatccttcgt ggacatcttc gtattgctgg acaccatcta ggacgctgtg
27001 acatcaagga cctgcctaaa gaaatcactg ttgctacatc acgaacgctt tcttattaca
27061 aattgggagc ttcgcagcgt gtagcaggtg actcaggttt tgctgcatac agtcgctaca
27121 ggattggcaa ctataaatta aacacagacc attccagtag cagtgacaat attgctttgc
27181 ttgtacagta agtgacaaca gatgtttcat ctcgttgact ttcaggttac tatagcagag
27241 atattactaa ttattatgag gacttttaaa gtttccattt ggaatcttga ttacatcata
27301 aacctcataa ttaaaaattt atctaagtca ctaactgaga ataaatattc tcaattagat
27361 gaagagcaac caatggagat tgattaaacg aacatgaaaa ttattctttt cttggcactg
27421 ataacactcg ctacttgtga gctttatcac taccaagagt gtgttagagg tacaacagta
27481 cttttaaaag aaccttgctc ttctggaaca tacgagggca attcaccatt tcatcctcta
27541 gctgataaca aatttgcact gacttgcttt agcactcaat ttgcttttgc ttgtcctgac
27601 ggcgtaaaac acgtctatca gttacgtgcc agatcagttt cacctaaact gttcatcaga
27661 caagaggaag ttcaagaact ttactctcca atttttctta ttgttgcggc aatagtgttt
27721 ataacacttt gcttcacact caaaagaaag acagaatgat tgaactttca ttaattgact
27781 tctatttgtg cttttagcc tttctgctat tccttgtttt aattatgctt attatctttt
27841 ggttctcact tgaactgcaa gatcataatg aaacttgtca cgcctaaacg aacatgaaat
27901 ttcttgtttt cttaggaatc atcacaactg tagctgcatt tcaccaagaa tgtagtttac
27961 agtcatgtac tcaacatcaa ccatatgtag ttgatgaccc gtgtcctatt cacttctatt
28021 ctaaatggta tattagagta ggagctagaa aatcagcacc tttaattgaa ttgtgcgtgg
28081 atgaggctgg ttctaaatca cccattcagt acatcgatat cggtaattat acagtttcct
28141 gtttaccttt tacaattaat tgccaggaac ctaaattggg tagtcttgta gtgcgttgtt
28201 cgttctatga agactttta gagtatcatg acgttcgtgt tgttttagat ttcatctaaa
28261 cgaacaaact aaaatgtctg ataatggacc ccaaaatcag cgaaatgcac cccgcattac
28321 gtttggtgga cccctcagatt caactggcag taaccagaat ggagaacgca gtgggggcgcg
28381 atcaaaacaa cgtcggcccc aaggtttacc caataatact gcgtcttggt tcaccgctct
28441 cactcaacat ggcaaggaag accttaaatt ccctcgagga caaggcgttc caattaacac
28501 caatagcagt ccagatgacc aaattggcta ctaccgaaga gctaccagac gaattcgtgg
28561 tggtgacggt aaaatgaaag atctcagtcc aagatggtat ttctactacc taggaactgg
28621 gccagaagct ggacttccct atggtgctaa caaagacggc atcatatggg ttgcaactga
28681 gggagccttg aatacaccaa aagatcacat tggcacccgc aatcctgcta caatgctgc
28741 aatcgtgcta caacttcctc aaggaacaac attgccaaaa ggcttctacg cagaagggag
28801 cagaggcggc agtcaagcct cttctcgttc ctcatcacgt agtcgcaaca gttcaagaaa
28861 ttcaactcca ggcagcagta ggggaacttc tcctgctaga atggctggca atggcggtga
28921 tgctgctctt gctttgctgc tgcttgacag attgaaccag cttgagagca aaatgtctgg
28981 taaaggccaa caacaacaag gccaaactgt cactaagaaa tctgctgctg aggcttctaa
29041 gaagcctcgg caaaaacgta ctgccactaa agcatacaat gtaacacaag ctttcggcag
```

89

```
29101  acgtggtcca gaacaaaccc aaggaaattt tggggaccag gaactaatca gacaaggaac
29161  tgattacaaa cattggccgc aaattgcaca atttgccccc agcgcttcag cgttcttcgg
29221  aatgtcgcgc attggcatgg aagtcacacc ttcgggaacg tggttgacct acacaggtgc
29281  catcaaattg gatgacaaag atccaaattt caaagatcaa gtcatttgc tgaataagca
29341  tattgacgca tacaaaacat tcccaccaac agagcctaaa aaggacaaaa agaagaaggc
29401  tgatgaaact caagccttac cgcagagaca gaagaaacag caaactgtga ctcttcttcc
29461  tgctgcagat ttggatgatt tctccaaaca attgcaacaa tccatgagca gtgctgactc
29521  aactcaggcc taaactcatg cagaccacac aaggcagatg gctatataa acgttttcgc
29581  ttttccgttt acgatatata gtctactctt gtgcagaatg aattctcgta actacatagc
29641  acaagtagat gtagttaact ttaatctcac atagcaatct ttaatcagtg tgtaacatta
29701  gggaggactt gaaagagcca ccacattttc accgaggcca cgcggagtac gatcgagtgt
29761  acagtgaaca atgctaggga gagctgccta tatggaagag ccctaatgtg taaaattaat
29821  tttagtagtg ctatcccat gtgattttaa tagcttctta ggagaatgac aaaaaaaaaa
29881  aaaaaaaaaa aaaaaaaaaa aaa
```

## Spike protein amino acid sequence

```
         10         20         30         40         50
MFIFLLFLTL TSGSDLDRCT TFDDVQAPNY TQHTSSMRGV YYPDEIFRSD
         60         70         80         90        100
TLYLTQDLFL PFYSNVTGFH TINHTFGNPV IPFKDGIYFA ATEKSNVVRG
        110        120        130        140        150
WVFGSTMNNK SQSVIIINNS TNVVIRACNF ELCDNPFFAV SKPMGTQTHT
        160        170        180        190        200
MIFDNAFNCT FEYISDAFSL DVSEKSGNFK HLREFVFKNK DGFLYVYKGY
        210        220        230        240        250
QPIDVVRDLP SGFNTLKPIF KLPLGINITN FRAILTAFSP AQDIWGTSAA
        260        270        280        290        300
AYFVGYLKPT TFMLKYDENG TITDAVDCSQ NPLAELKCSV KSFEIDKGIY
        310        320        330        340        350
QTSNFRVVPS GDVVRFPNIT NLCPFGEVFN ATKFPSVYAW ERKKISNCVA
        360        370        380        390        400
DYSVLYNSTF FSTFKCYGVS ATKLNDLCFS NVYADSFVVK GDDVRQIAPG
        410        420        430        440        450
QTGVIADYNY KLPDDFMGCV LAWNTRNIDA TSTGNYNYKY RYLRHGKLRP
        460        470        480        490        500
FERDISNVPF SPDGKPCTPP ALNCYWPLND YGFYTTTGIG YQPYRVVVLS
        510        520        530        540        550
FELLNAPATV CGPKLSTDLI KNQCVNFNFN GLTGTGVLTP SSKRFQPFQQ
        560        570        580        590        600
FGRDVSDFTD SVRDPKTSEI LDISPCSFGG VSVITPGTNA SSEVAVLYQD
        610        620        630        640        650
VNCTDVSTAI HADQLTPAWR IYSTGNNVFQ TQAGCLIGAE HVDTSYECDI
        660        670        680        690        700
PIGAGICASY HTVSLLRSTS QKSIVAYTMS LGADSSIAYS NNTIAIPTNF
        710        720        730        740        750
SISITTEVMP VSMAKTSVDC NMYICGDSTE CANLLLQYGS FCTQLNRALS
        760        770        780        790        800
GIAAEQDRNT REVFAQVKQM YKTPTLKYFG GFNFSQILPD PLKPTKRSFI
        810        820        830        840        850
EDLLFNKVTL ADAGFMKQYG ECLGDINARD LICAQKFNGL TVLPPLLTDD
        860        870        880        890        900
MIAAYTAALV SGTATAGWTF GAGAALQIPF AMQMAYRFNG IGVTQNVLYE
        910        920        930        940        950
NQKQIANQFN KAISQIQESL TTTSTALGKL QDVVNQNAQA LNTLVKQLSS
        960        970        980        990       1000
NFGAISSVLN DILSRLDKVE AEVQIDRLIT GRLQSLQTYV TQQLIRAAEI
       1010       1020       1030       1040       1050
RASANLAATK MSECVLGQSK RVDFCGKGYH LMSFPQAAPH GVVFLHVTYV
       1060       1070       1080       1090       1100
PSQERNFTTA PAICHEGKAY FPREGVFVFN GTSWFITQRN FFSPQIITTD
```

```
          1110       1120       1130       1140       1150
     NTFVSGNCDV VIGIINNTVY DPLQPELDSF KEELDKYFKN HTSPDVDLGD
          1160       1170       1180       1190       1200
     ISGINASVVN IQKEIDRLNE VAKNLNESLI DLQELGKYEQ YIKWPWYVWL
          1210       1220       1230       1240       1250
     GFIAGLIAIV MVTILLCCMT SCCSCLKGAC SCGSCCKFDE DDSEPVLKGV

     KLHYT
```